Crystal

Health &
Happiness
:)
Angela

The Glucometer: A Self-Empowering Tool to a Healthy and Lean Body

A.M. Ross

Edits by Ms. Molly McKitterick, The Word Process, Washington, D.C.

authorHOUSE®

AuthorHouse™
1663 Liberty Drive
Bloomington, IN 47403
www.authorhouse.com
Phone: 1-800-839-8640

Published by AuthorHouse   4/20/2012

ISBN: 978-1-4685-7631-3 (sc)
ISBN: 978-1-4685-7982-6 (e)

Library of Congress Control Number: 2012906600

For my daughters, Sydney Nikole and Rachel Kharin Ross, I wish for you to always remain a work in progress. I pray you never forget to just BE you. The most amazing thing you will ever do is to fully explore who you are. Never struggle to fit into parameters established by others. Be loud, silly, tender, loving, fun, awkward and wonderful. You will be the best YOU when you listen closely to the spirit of Sydney or Rachel. Helping create, nurture and teach you both is hands down the most beautiful, strong thing I have accomplished. I love you both.

The Glucometer: A Self-Empowering Tool to a Healthy and Lean Body

Introduction

For the first time in my life I am not worried about my weight, or my body fat percentage.

When I look in the mirror, I am happy with the person staring back. That's a bold statement considering I have been chasing the perfect body since I was eleven years old. I have arrived at this happy place thanks to a glucometer. What is a glucometer? It is a home medical testing device used to determine the concentration of glucose in your blood.

I am not diabetic. I don't need to test my blood glucose levels for medical reasons. But after months of testing myself, I can tell you that it is impossible to know how a food impacts your health and how much unsightly body fat that food can cause you to accumulate without the glucometer. Unless you are aware of what is going on inside your body, food choices, even choices you think are good for you, can be a health blind spot – a health blind spot that can be absolved with a speck of blood and a glucometer.

I have a Bachelors of Science degree in Health and Sports Science. In addition, I have certifications as a personal trainer, group fitness instructor, performance enhancement specialist and performance nutrition with Aerobic and Fitness Association of America (AFAA), National Exercise Trainers Association (formerly, NDEITA) and National Academy of Sports Medicine (NASM).

I completed over thirty physical fitness tests (PFTs) for the Marine Corps with an Iron Woman status (Iron Man/Woman status is scoring 285 points or higher out of a total of 300 points on a range of physical tests). I have competed in figure competitions, I ran a competitive marathon, and I've done the Tough Mudder, fitness competitions and aerobic marathons.

For eight years, I have been a Personal Trainer, coaching and educating clients. I have experience training amateur athletes and college football players, as well as individuals with diabetes and heart conditions. I have trained Marines, cops, house moms and desk jockeys.

My personal expertise and favorite aspect of training is in nutrition. For years, I experimented and refined the details of my personal diet to create a complete, thorough and effective program for *you*. This program is the *lifestyle* that I advise for my clients. The lifestyle that had a woman abandon medications she had taken for seven years to treat her high blood pressure. A lifestyle that has cured the symptoms of endometriosis, quieted Rheumatoid arthritis, identified Celiac Disease symptoms and lose accumulated fat.

One of the top requests I get from clients is 'just tell me what to eat'. This is an impossible request. If a trainer designs a program for you and dictates your meals and you don't want chicken for dinner or fish for lunch, you feel as if you are failing the program. Here is where the glucometer can help. The glucometer will guide you in your food choices and help you determine the best foods for you and timing of those foods to be healthy and lean

In this book, I am including recipes, grocery lists, daily challenges, and an exercise program that can be tailored to fit your needs. You will develop your own menu and workouts at your current gym or in your own home with as little or as much equipment as you decide.

Imagine a lifestyle program that incorporates what is really important about diet and exercise *without gimmicks*: no shake weights, abs rollers, horses, or lounges. No fancy, expensive shakes or caffeine laced pills. This is a program for *real* people with careers, kids; busy lives.

My program isn't just about losing weight. It is designed to help you obtain optimal health and longevity. This is you taking control of you through the management of your blood glucose levels, using food, exercise and the glucometer. *FOOD IS THE MOST POWERFUL MEDICINE.* Hippocrates said "Let food be your medicine and medicine be your food." This should be the cornerstone of your health because when you are healthy, you are lean.

The program's goal is for *you* to prioritize *your* health. Will it work? That is a question only *you* can answer. Your time is the most valuable thing you have. I ask you to give me a **concentrated effort** for three weeks to see a difference, a 100 percent dedication and devotion to the program. The effectiveness of this program, *if you dedicate yourself to it*, is so absolute, three weeks could change the quality of your life.

I promised you no gimmicks. A healthy and lean body requires work. Motivation is what will get you started, but habit is what will keep you going. Habits are still choices and you will have to make the right choice each day. With the use of a glucometer, you will have the appropriate information to get you healthy and lean, no more guessing.

Your goal, while following this program, is to obtain and maintain consistent blood glucose levels between 80-90 milligrams/deciliter (mg/dl). To help you achieve this I have laid out a plan with the important times to test your blood glucose levels for the data you need to determine what to eat. I have also developed exercise routines in a 21-day journal format.

This is the complete plan for your success: exciting and tasty recipes, grocery lists, treats, exercise plans, how to make your own exercise equipment, stretches, how to determine if you have mobility issues and correct them to prevent injuries, a journal and fasts.

Chapter One:

Why I designed this program?

I am not a doctor. I have never been to medical school. All of the knowledge I have is from self-experimentation and education, and through the kindness of my family and friends who let me experiment on them. They are real people with real jobs and obstacles just like you that include taxiing kids to extra-curricular activities, long commutes, house work, pets, work travel and any emotional struggles you can think of.

A little background on me, I am a former Marine. I was active duty in the Marine Corps from 1998-2006. I currently work fulltime as a Department of Defense employee in Washington, DC. I have a crazy commute and work long hours. I am a cop's wife, and we have two daughters: Sydney, 12 and Rachel, 10.

At the age of fifteen, I started weight lifting with a trainer who was in his seventies and had done bodybuilding shows. At seventy, he was in better shape than the kids my age. At the time, I wanted to be a Coast Guard rescue swimmer. I trained hard every single day. I absorbed everything he had to teach me. His work ethic was, when you are here you train hard. He didn't want excuses, and he didn't want to hear complaints. He was selective about his clientele, and I was very lucky to be on the list. I didn't want to get fired!

Back then, I had no idea how to eat properly and lived largely off peanut butter on bread and milk.

At the request of my mother, I didn't join the Coast Guard and went off to college. I joined a gym close to school and was exposed to more body builders and what became iconic to me….the figure girls. One woman in particular, Sharon, was like a unicorn, beautiful and majestic. She had the perfect tan and make-up and the best workout clothes. All the guys at the gym wanted to date her; and all the girls wanted her advice on training. Her muscular figure was feminine, and her fake boobs were perky. I decided right then and there, that was what I wanted to look like. I wanted be a figure competitor.

I was taking advice from any bodybuilder at the gym who would talk to me. Being young and naive, I tried to follow all the advice from the good to the bad to the questionable. Because I was still new to weight lifting, I was making some muscle gains, but I wasn't looking like Sharon fast enough! The head trainer, Jamie – also Sharon's boyfriend – was extremely helpful on my quest to figure fame. He leant me books on Olympic lifting and helped me tweak my diet. I lived on microwaveable chicken breasts that I dipped in spaghetti sauce and protein shakes during my sixteen months at school.

After college, I went back to Altoona, PA and started working at a Holiday Inn as a front desk clerk. I supplemented my little income with waitressing at Pizza Hut. Low and behold this wasn't the life I wanted to lead. I signed up and shipped off to the Marine Corps. Sorry mom.

My years in the Marine Corps brought me a whole new base for fitness. We took bi-annual physical fitness tests (PFT) that consisted of a three-mile run, flexed-arm hangs for the women and pull-ups for the men, and timed crunches. My main focus was to be better than the men. There is a certain stigma about females in the Corps, and I wasn't going to embody it. If the boys were doing pull-ups, then I was doing pull-ups. If the boys were running hard and fast, than I was running hard and fast. I didn't want any gender leniency. I wanted to be as good as the men, and I wanted the men who weren't good to be ashamed.

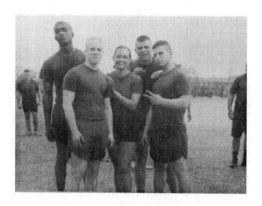

Camp Lejeune, NC 2001

Although slender, my body was far from lean and muscular like Sharon's. In 2002, after I had my second daughter, the spark to be a figure girl was rekindled, and I started training hard to get on stage.

I immersed myself in popular bodybuilding websites and forums. I read blog journals of girls who had been successful on stage and those that were, like me, on the current journey. There is a plethora of information out there.

During my competition prep, I went from 132 pounds and twenty percent body fat to 118 pounds and twelve percent body fat. I wasn't well prepared and hardly had any muscle to display. The advice I got from the judges after the show was to bulk, put on more muscle, and try again.

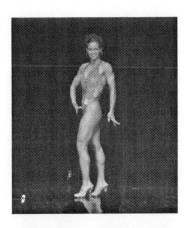

Angela on stage, NGA Competition

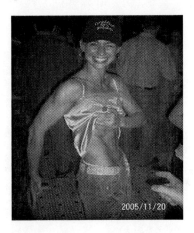

Celebrating after the show, November, 2005

This was a frightening concept to me. They were asking me to put on a bunch of weight, inevitably some would be fat, hopefully most muscle, then diet back down and see where I was. Determined to be a unicorn, I decided to give it a try.

My one and only attempt at a bulk went like this: no cardio, only heavy Olympic lifts. Pre-workout, I drank amped up pre-work out supplements; mid-workout, I ate some sweet tarts and a protein gel shot drink; post-work out, I had a protein drink. I got stronger on my lifts. I put on some noticeable size and was weighing in at about 144 pounds. None of my clothes fit, and I couldn't do a flight of stairs without becoming winded. My legs were ham hocks; my shoulders had a nice cap to them; my face was round; and my triceps puffy. Did I mention my clothes didn't fit?

To top it all off, I kept getting injured. These were relative changes – depends on who views them as to if they were good or bad. I viewed them as "things you learn as you get older in the gym" and I will never do any of this crap again.

The supplements I was drinking were tearing up my stomach. I was bloated, my stomach ached, and I had horrible gas. Any type of powdered mix, whether it was the caffeine amped pre-work out drinks (containing caffeine, B-6, sucralose, aspirin and a ton of other chemicals), or a protein powder (containing whey, vitamins and minerals and artificial sweeteners) has to be mixed with water. I used as little water as possible (the suggested amount was eight ounces of water, I was using about two ounces) to gag them down and then rubbed my belly like a Buddha to try to get it to stop reeling. I routinely got pimples on my back and face.

I became chronically constipated with intermittent periods of blasting diarrhea. On one specific day, I had spent the morning and early afternoon at a playground with my daughters. On the drive home, we were hitting every traffic light possible. I was getting nauseous and could feel the bout of diarrhea ascending my poor abused colon. In the car, there wasn't much I could do but pray I'd make it home in time. Unfortunately, I only made it to the front door. Try explaining to your three year old that they shouldn't poop in their pants when mommy is doing it.

Did I mention my clothes didn't fit? In addition to all the fake sugars and chemicals that were in the supplements (and supments are 'spensive!), I drank diet cola, put Splenda on/in everything, ate sugar free Jell-O, sugar free chocolates, and invented a sugar free pumpkin pie. (My sugar free pumpkin pie invention almost got me divorced; according to my husband's rule book you don't mess with pumpkin pie!) The only other things I was eating were grilled chicken and green beans. I wouldn't eat steak to prevent high cholesterol and excessive weight gain. I was always hungry and had nicknamed my hunger "my inner fat girl." This is sadly ironic because I was becoming fat on the outside as my body fat crawled into the 20% and over range. I cringed….but I was bulking, I kept telling myself.

I finally came to my senses and stopped tormenting my digestive system. I stopped eating all non-foods (all my wonderful fake sugar creations). I adopted what I coined "clean eating." Clean eating was basically grilled chicken; rotisserie turkey as well as turkey bacon, burger and pepperoni; green beans, spinach and broccoli; low-carb Breads; plain Greek yogurts with Polaner's All Fruit; hummus and pita chips; brown and yellow rice; garbanzo beans and lentils; and lots of fruit. Although I was feeling better I still battled chronic constipation and acne breakouts. I chalked it up to bad genetics and marched on.

I finished my Bachelor's degree in Health and Sports Science. I hadn't learned much from college about training or coaching so I researched the best certifications for personal training and obtained them. I studied to be a personal trainer, group fitness instructor, performance enhancement specialist and performance nutrition with Aerobic and Fitness Association of America (AFAA), National Exercise Trainers Association (formerly NDEITA) and National Academy of Sports Medicine (NASM).

In 2003, I started taking clients as a personal trainer and instructing a boot-camp style class on the base I was stationed. In 2006, I got out of the Marine Corps and started a business doing in-home personal training. I would go to a client's home with all the equipment, walk them through a workout and give them nutritional guidance. I loved doing it, but the summer brought sky rocketing gas prices and I wasn't making enough money to pay the mortgage and feed the kids, so I got my current job at the Defense Department. My DoD job pays the bills, but I continue to take clients on the side so that I can continue to do what I love most: help people transform their lives.

I am not a fan of the term "personal trainer." There are many more personal trainers with too little knowledge and experience than there are really great ones. And this is a shame. A great personal trainer will transform your life, not just your body. I coach my clients to be a better person in every aspect. My motto is a strong mind, a strong body. One of the most important things I have learned from working with people over the last nine years is that your life has to be complete to be healthy. All the pieces have to be in place.

Some days, I am that bitch yelling and screaming at clients to work harder and move faster through a workout. The next day, I am encouraging proper form. The next, I may be talking with them about difficulties with an unsupportive spouse or post-partum depression. I am a cheerleader, a towel holder, a psychologist, and an exercise coach. Everything that my clients go through when they are outside of my gym affects their progress. The magic that happens in my gym is only fifteen percent of the solution to health and a lean body. That fact has to be acknowledged and addressed by a trainer.

I am summing up my eighteen years of experience in a few short pages, but this isn't an autobiography, and this book isn't about me. It's about you and how you will apply and benefit from the information I researched, tested and continue to practice.

Chapter Two:

Glucose Levels, Insulin and Disease

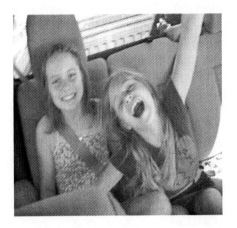

Sydney and Rachel

Celiac Disease

My youngest daughter, Rachel, was diagnosed with Celiac in December, 2010. Celiac Disease is an autoimmune disease. Symptoms for Rachel include severe fatigue, bad stomach pains, and rashes. She was severely underweight.

Celiac Disease is a condition that damages the lining of the small intestine and prevents it from absorbing parts of food that are important for staying healthy. The damage is due to a reaction to eating gluten and inability to tolerate gluten. Gluten is the protein found in grains.

The cure for Rachel was to cut out all wheat and other gluten-bearing grains from her diet. I was making "special" bread for her that consisted of a lot of chemicals and rice flour which she didn't like. I made pancake mixes made with a lot of chemicals, rice flour and potato starch which she didn't like. She also didn't like gluten free brownies, cookies, pizza and macaroni. I jumped through hoops to try and accommodate her as a "kid" so she could eat "normal" and still "enjoy her life."

I was looking at the situation wrongly. Rachel's Celiac was making her sick and not letting her be a "normal kid" or "enjoy her life". It had her so sick she couldn't get off the couch to play with a friend she had invited over to play. She hadn't gained any weight in several years (at eight years old she was forty-four pounds, the same weight she had been at four years old) and was very frail in appearance. Being unable to play because you are too sick and being frighteningly underweight is not normal or enjoying life. Her body, as everyone's does, needed **real** foods, with nutrients that would allow her to grow strong, vibrant and be healthy.

The medical community wasn't any help. I was told she could have wheat as she could tolerate it. SHE COULDN'T TOLERATE IT!!! And because she had Celiac disease she was more susceptible to develop other autoimmune diseases like Type I Diabetes or Multiple Sclerosis. Another down side to Gluten Free foods is they are made of rice flour and potato starch which are powdered and crushed, no digestion required, so they immediately enter the blood stream and spike blood glucose levels even higher than grains and sugars, which is a fast track to diabetes. Gluten-free foods are the new "fat-free" for the food industry.

14

A Paleo Solution

I set out on a mission to educate myself on how to best feed my family with our new obstacle. Our family is a united family. If Rachel wasn't able to have foods made with grains, then none of us were going to have them. After extensive research my family went "Paleo."

The Paleo diet is in simple terms eating like a caveman. Robb Wolf does a much better job of explaining the Paleo diet in his book, and I definitely recommend reading *The Paleo Diet Solution*. Not only does he tell a great story but he is a bio-chemist and explains in great, well researched details the negative effect grains will have on your health. It's a well written book.

About six months into the Paleo lifestyle; which discourages eating the following: grains, legumes (to include peanuts) and their oils, dairy, starchy tubers, sugars, processed meats, and corn oil; I started missing certain foods in my diet. I like heavy whipping cream in my coffee; I like bacon and sausage (nitrate-free though); Greek yogurt; I also like potatoes and rice. I don't have potatoes or rice often.

But I love heavy whipping cream in my coffee every day, and if we are being realistic, it's more like three times a day. I may even have bacon or sausage every day. My favorite post-workout meal is plain Greek yogurt.

I do agree with the Paleo lifestyle in that the quality of your food is of utmost importance. For instance, my Greek yogurt and heavy whipping cream brands have been researched to ensure that recombinant bovine somatotropin (rBST), a synthetic hormone given to cows to increase milk production is not used. The Food and Drug Administration does not require genetically engineered foods to be labeled so it is a daunting task, but one well worth it. There have been no long term studies on the effects of rBST on humans, but in cows it causes cancerous tumors. I believe rBST raises estrogen levels in both men and women.

We need to pay attention to what they are feeding, and how the animals we consume are treated. The urban legend of how the Human Immunodeficiency Virus (HIV) was started is a great example of why you should care. Rumors gave HIV's origins the tale of Zoophilia with an African monkey; however HIV was spread to mankind by EATING the African monkeys. Food for thought?

At the same time as I was missing my non-Paleo foods, I started to explore the body's hormonal homeostasis and the importance of the hormone, insulin, and its important impact on blood glucose levels and the negative effects of having blood glucose levels over 100 mg/dl. An ideal blood glucose reading is 80-90 mg/dl, roughly 60-90 minutes after a meal. I started testing my blood glucose levels pre and post meals and then experimented with certain foods that were "non-Paleo" to see how my blood glucose levels tolerated them.

I could not tolerate wheat, sugars, or beans. They spiked my blood glucose levels and messed up my stomach. And maintaining a blood glucose level of 80-90 mg/dl, ninety minutes after eating was what had become most important to me.

I started to feel a little guilty about my Paleo disloyalty. The Paleo lifestyle had helped my family in a tremendous way. My daughter was healthy, my husband had lost weight, and I wasn't having any digestive issues. The pressure of staying with it was starting to deteriorate my spirits, and I was having self-doubt about my skills to help other people. I mean if I couldn't follow this lifestyle I could not instruct others to.

My saving grace was my love for the Paleo Diet had sparked my interest in Evolution and Anthropology. My Anthropology studies led me to discover our ancestors were in BETTER SHAPE, BETTER HEALTH, and had blood glucose levels between 80-90 mg/dl. *And* that is what *all* mammals are supposed to have for optimal health. This intrigued me and I started down the path of hormones, insulin in particular, and their impact on our health and weight loss ability.

One of the key hormones in our body that determines health and how lean we are is *insulin*. Insulin regulates the amount of glucose in the blood. Any more than five grams of glucose in the blood is toxic and the body will work very hard to remove that glucose from the blood stream. *Carbohydrates* in any form, except fiber, start to turn to glucose *as soon* as they hit your tongue.

Our primitive ancestors ate about twenty-two teaspoons of sugar per year, mostly in the form of honey and fruit, which is seasonal in most areas. The honey and the sugar had to be foraged, and hunting for it burned most of the sugar they consumed immediately. Today, Americans average about sixty teaspoons of sugar a day, and the most foraging done is the walk from the office desk to the vending machine.

Insulin

Insulin is a chemical messenger that directs cellular activities; if your insulin is out of whack, you can diet and exercise until you drop without success. Your cells *have* to hear the correct signal. If your cells are getting the right message, then you will lose more with less exercise.

The pancreas produces insulin to sweep the glucose out of the blood and stores it in the muscle tissues. If those muscles are full, the excess glucose is stored as fat. This stored fat accumulates in the organs (which is called visceral fat) or accumulates on the butt and triceps (harmless but unsightly). Where fat is stored depends largely on genetics.

Glucose levels consistently higher than 100 mg/dl can result in harmless but unsightly fat that hugs the butt, flaps around the triceps, or doubles the chin. It also creates dangerous and metabolically active, visceral fat. Visceral fat is the fat that accumulates in the liver, the kidneys, the heart, the pancreas and the intestines and is seen on the body as the coined term "muffin top" (fat that hangs over the waist line of pants or skirts) and belly fat.

Blood glucose levels are affected by a variety of factors like the foods we eat, any beverages other than water, infection, alcohol and stress.

Infection is a common cause of high blood glucose levels. Any type of illness, infection, surgery, dental problem, injury and even emotional stress will cause stress on the body. Your body needs more energy to battle these stressors and will produce hormones that tell the liver to release extra glucose to provide that energy.

The production of these hormones inhibits the effectiveness of insulin and as a result, the blood glucose level rises.

In late July last year, my blood glucose levels were reading high. I ate a burger wrapped in lettuce with avocado and broccoli and got a 90 minute post meal reading of 174. I was freaking out! Why was my blood glucose level reading so high? The next morning, I woke up with severe congestion and what progressed into the worst sinus infection I have ever had.

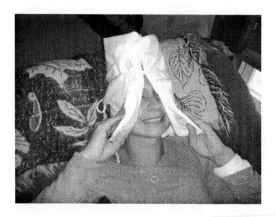

Trying to alleviate my sinus pressure with a heat pad

I called my sister-in-law and asked if my nephew, who has Type I diabetes, has trouble with his blood glucose levels when he is sick. She told me that when he gets sick his glucose levels are uncontrollable. This explained to me why my readings were high leading up to and during my sinus infection.

After my sinus infection was gone and I felt better, my readings were still on the high side. Not as high as they had been as the infection was coming on and during, but still too high. I began to research how long diabetics blood glucose levels are high after an infection and didn't find any concrete information. I did read that red blood cells have a 100-120 day life span. Once a glucose molecule attaches itself to a red blood cell it persists for the life of that red blood cell. This meant my levels were going to be on the higher side until the life span of the red blood cells, which had been around for my sinus infection, was over.

This was an eye opening experience for me. In the past if my daughters or I had an upset stomach, we would drink a ginger ale soda to help us feel better.

Or if I was getting a cold and just felt like eating junk, I would give myself the "sick pass." But this is detrimental to health! Your glucose blood levels are already elevated, and drinking a soda for an upset stomach during the flu or giving yourself the "sick pass" to eat junk food is spiking your glucose levels even higher and making your pancreas and other organs work even harder!!

The best remedy for infections is lots of water to stay hydrated, lots of rest to give your body the ability to focus on fighting the infection, and eating as little as possible only fat and protein centered foods.

The last big impact on insulin is alcohol. Alcohol should be consumed in extreme moderation. It is considered poison by the body, and all efforts are made to expel it, including the interruption of maintaining healthy blood glucose levels. Over time, excessive alcohol consumption can decrease insulin's effectiveness, resulting in high blood sugar levels. Alcohol consumption should be saved for celebrations; it truly is a hindrance on your health.

There are numerous articles on the benefits of red wine and anti-oxidants. However the actual study is extremely unclear on the amount of red wine that is considered "good"; and the health benefits of red wine come from the skin of the grapes used to make the wine. You can eat grapes for these antioxidants rather than drinking red wine, providing you the benefits without taking the chance of over doing it with alcohol.

Visceral Fat

Visceral fat is metabolically active fat that causes chronic (meaning constant) inflammation. Chronic inflammation leads to heart disease, diabetes, high blood pressure, sleep apnea, stroke, cancer and a number of degenerative diseases. This is why visceral fat is dangerous and not just unsightly in a Speedo or pouring over the top of skinny jeans.

The unsightly fat that you see on your belly is only the visible problem. The fat that you can't see is the dangerous, visceral fat. Fat deposits accumulate around and within, internal organs such as the liver, and when the liver gets fat, it becomes more insulin resistant. A fatty liver is told to produce more glucose than needed, raising blood sugar and causing a further rise in insulin. This is a vicious cycle resulting in more insulin resistance.

When the liver is full of fat, then fat is sent to be stored in the arteries, which increases risk of heart attack.

Are you beginning to see the relationship between insulin and the common, widespread diseases affecting our population? This fat accumulation is the catalyst for obesity, diabetes, heart disease, and early death.

If your metabolism (metabolism is the body's *whole* hormonal response to processing food and energy production) has to produce large amounts of insulin (insulin is the master hormone of the metabolism) to sweep the excess glucose (anything over that five grams is toxic) out of your blood stream consistently, the fat burning "mechanism" (your cells not getting the correct message from insulin) will turn off, and fat will accumulate. An onslaught of deadly problems may follow to include: heart disease, hardening of the arteries, damage to the artery walls, increased cholesterol levels, vitamins and mineral deficiencies, and kidney disease.

Too Much Insulin is Dangerous

Let's talk pancreas. The pancreas has both alpha-cells and beta-cells; your beta-cells are where the hormone insulin, is produced.

We have two insulin responses to mopping excess glucose from the blood. The first response is called the *initial response*. The amount of insulin released in this initial response is based directly on your last meal. If this initial response isn't effective at returning your blood glucose levels to under 90 mg/dl, your body will put into effect the second phase, which is called the *insulin response*. The insulin response will continue to pump insulin in an attempt to regulate glucose levels to under 90 mg/dl. This is an extremely *oversimplified* explanation of a very complex function; but it allows you to easily see how the beta-cells in your pancreas can be worked overtime if you are on a carbohydrate based diet, especially if you more than you should and don't get any exercise, which cause large amounts of glucose to be dumped into your blood stream.

The real problem starts when these precious beta-cells start to die from overuse. Yep, that's right; your beta-cells are not replenishable. Once their lifespan is up; that's the end for them. When sixty-three percent of your beta-cells die, you are considered a diabetic. Unfortunately, there is no test to count beta-cells in a living human.

A biopsy would cause the pancreas to leak digestive enzymes, and digestive enzymes would do just what they are designed to do: digest, even if it is pancreas tissue. This is obviously no good.

An MRI cannot be used because of the location of the pancreas. There is research being done now on beta-cell regeneration and there are projects in the works to convert adult pancreas alpha-cells' function to beta-cell function to replace dead beta-cells. But it is in the very infant stages.

The best protection is prevention. Treating symptoms with medication only masks the problem, and it will eventually get worse or the medication will have side effects that cause additional complications. Medication is not a cure; it is a treatment. Reducing or eliminating foods that cause unnecessary glucose spikes and exercise are the best preventive measures to keeping your pancreas healthy. Maintaining blood glucose levels of 80-90 mg/dl prevents heart disease, high blood pressure, cancers and degenerative diseases.

Blood glucose levels are commonly monitored for the diagnosis of diabetes. You are probably aware that there are two types of diabetes: Type I and Type II.

Type 1 in simple terms occurs when the pancreas doesn't make insulin.

Type 2 in simple terms is when the pancreas is makes too much insulin and the tissues and cells become insulin resistant – they no longer respond to this hormone. Insulin is a yellin' and screamin' – but your tissues aren't a listenin'. Your body is making enough insulin to control blood glucose levels; however your cells don't know how to use it effectively or efficiently. And, as discussed, if your cells aren't receiving the right messages, then you will start to accumulate fat and get sick.

By monitoring your blood glucose levels and maintaining them at 80-90 mg/dl you can not only prevent diabetes and the laundry list of other diseases, but you can get lean. How do you monitor and maintain blood glucose levels? Keep reading!

Chapter Three:

Removing the Barriers to a Healthy Lifestyle

<u>Fasting</u>

I completely understand the initial knee jerk reaction to fasting, can be frightening. We associate fasting with medical tests, being hungry and muscle wasting. We are socialized to think fasting will cause the wasting of our muscle tissue from years of nutritionists prompting us to eat every 2-3 hours or eat 5-6 small meals a day.

Where does a fast fit into this sound advice? That's the problem. It is *not* sound advice. Most personal trainers, nutritionists and even registered dieticians recommend eating every 2-3 hours or 5-6 small meals, a technique to offer food discipline. The problem with this technique is the mechanics of it are flawed.

 A typical case is Jane. Jane wakes up. In a hurry, she skips breakfast, drops the kids at daycare, and heads to work. Jane is short on time during her lunch break because of her workload and can't leave her desk for more than a few minutes. She didn't pack anything so she buys a bag of chips and a soda out of the vending machine to eat at her desk. An hour later, she is starving, but there is no time to eat among finishing her work day, her commute home, getting the kids from school and a number of errands that must be completed. Jane is a typical, busy, working mom. Jane finally gets home and is so hungry that she makes horrible food choices (microwavable frozen foods, chips, and the like) and over eats.

After reviewing Jane's dietary habits, her nutritionist suggests she go to the common five – six meals a day plan. The nutritionist has her add a quick breakfast shake, and then, pack fruit and nuts for an early morning snack, a sensible lunch, and another snack of fruit and nuts for the ride home. At home, she should eat a healthy dinner. Her nutritionist recommends her dinner and lunch choices are whole grains, beans, dairy and lean proteins. This seems reasonable, right? This should set Jane up to control her hunger so that she can make better food choices, right? Wrong! And here is why.

Jane's hunger is a symptom from her poor diet choices and the spark of the "glucose hunger monster". A diet based on carbohydrates sets you up metabolically to be a glucose burner. When your body relies on glucose as its main source of energy – and all carbohydrates turn into glucose as soon as they hit your lips (did I mention this yet?) – you will always be hungry so as not to interrupt the energy supply. The blood, remember, can only hold five grams of sugar at a time. More than that and you start to target your muscle tissue and even bones for glucose fuel. Cannibalizing your own muscle and bone tissue for glucose is catabolism, and your body *IS* smart, it would rather *NOT* cannibalize itself. As a result, your brain will signal for food by causing fatigue, anxiety, irritability, explosive anger, jitters and more cravings. You can suffer energy loss, reduced mental and physical performance and you will have more carbohydrate cravings. The quality of your moods and thinking are often hugely dependent upon that steady supply of fuel. Carbohydrates are like rocket fuel; hot and fast.

Following this program will switch you from a sugar/glucose burner to a fat burner. As a fat burner eating becomes a choice rather than a constant necessity. Energy levels are maintained which allows for clearer thinking and a stable mood.

As a fat burner, you use ketones as fuel versus glucose. Ketones are energy units of fat. The big difference between ketones as fuel versus glucose is that ketones fuel is longer, better, more consistent, and reliable.

Using ketones as fuel is called ketosis. You may have heard that ketosis is dangerous. Ketosis is the result of the body manufacturing its own glucose to prevent low blood sugar and it is not dangerous. The term you may be thinking of is ketoacidosis. This is a potentially life threatening complication of primarily Type I diabetes in which the body responds to a shortage on insulin by burning fatty acids and producing acidic ketone bodies that cause a variety of symptoms. Ketosis and ketoacidosis are two completely different metabolic processes which share only the same by-product, ketones, and unfortunately have similar names.

Ketones, or fat and protein, as your primary source of fuel will allow you to reap the rewards of a fast, maintain healthy blood glucose levels and shed body fat.

Getting back to fasting and why you should fast. Fasting has extreme benefits for your blood glucose levels. By fasting, you give your pancreas a rest and the chance to stabilize your blood glucose levels before dumping more food into your system to be digested and metabolized. You also achieve these additional positive effects: reduce blood pressure; reduce visceral fat (the fat that releases inflammatory signals and generates resistance to insulin which , in turn, causes your pancreas to create *more* and we've established this is *no good)*; and accelerate weight loss. You will gain a greater appreciation for the natural flavor of foods, and who doesn't want their food to taste better?

In my program, I employ a 16-hour and a 20-hour fast. Nothing too crazy! Do not get intimidated. When the fasts are introduced as a challenge, you will be ready!

In our primitive days when food was scarce, we developed a method to keep us alive through times of famine. Our bodies recognized there wasn't enough food to feed us, and our genes focused their attention on maintaining and repairing the body to be lean, healthy and disease free. Mother Nature must love us because generations later, we still have this ability to maintain and repair.

By the use of fasts, you can "trick" your body into turning these repair and maintenance genes on, and your body will work to keep you lean, healthy and disease free. However, when your blood glucose levels are too high from consuming carbohydrates, your body is not able to switch into the repair and maintain mode. If you have a carbohydrate-based diet you will have a very hard time fasting because you will be too hungry. It is very hard to ignore the hunger monster cries on a carbohydrate-based diet.

Fasting will help you identify the difference between your physical hunger and your mental, emotional hunger. A good way to determine between physical hunger and mental hunger is when you determine you are hungry and start to reach for a "snack" of fruit, nuts, or something much worse, like a 100 calorie snack pack of anything...shudder. Stop and ask yourself, "If I replaced this snack with chicken and broccoli would I still want to eat?" If you wouldn't eat the chicken and broccoli over the snack then you are emotionally hungry vice physically hungry. When you are physically hungry, any food will do. Emotional hunger cries for junk. Fasting helps you recognize and separate the two hungers and say no to emotional eating.

Even fruit and nuts can be excessive calories. Besides the excess calories, they are a feeble attempt to feed a hunger that has nothing to do with your nutritional needs.

Love

Our food choices reflect how we honor our bodies and the harmony we have within ourselves. Emotional hunger isn't eased by eating, and emotional eating complicates the situation. In addition to being upset about yourself and/or your life, you are upset about your food choices.

The root cause of emotional eating and hunger has to be addressed. In the Daily Challenges in the journal portion of this plan, I have included exercises to teach you to love yourself. This may seem silly, but you must realize that you have to love yourself, first and foremost, to be happy and healthy. Being unhealthy, whether consuming alcohol regularly, smoking cigarettes, not wearing your seat belt in the car, eating foods that you know are not good for you, or eating when you are not hungry, are signs of emotional distress. They can lead to fat accumulation and health problems.

Love Exercises will include writing a letter to tell yourself how proud you are, telling those close to you in your life *out loud* that *you* love *you* and how that impacts the relationship you have with them, creating a reflection board, and a reflection walk.

A reflection board and a reflection walk are similar. The board is a visible area of your home or work space that you hang "feel good about you" memorabilia. It can be a letter from your spouse or parent, a promotion or kudos letter from work, a picture from a vacation, anything that makes you smile and feel good.

The reflection walk is done as a walk alone so you can reflect and remember all the wonderful, special moments in your life and remind yourself that if you want to keep enjoying special moments, you have to take care of yourself. This includes exercising daily, eating real food, not overeating, drinking water, staying away from booze, avoiding junk food and life junk and getting proper rest. *YOU ARE THAT IMPORTANT!*

The most important time to do Love Exercises is when you are emotionally hungry, when you have identified that your hunger isn't physical and that you just want to snack. Engaging your mind with a task can divert you from emotional eating. But it would be a good idea to identify why you want to sabotage your health by eating in excess or making food choices you know are not good for you. Then, refuse to let yourself give in to that impulse.

Having a bad day at work, a crappy commute home or feeling stressed from too many demands shouldn't be excuses to eat a few chips. Those chips aren't going to solve your problems at work, fix your commute or lighten your demand load. Those chips *will* cause your glucose levels to spike, accumulate fat and add to your depression.

Telling someone in your life that you love yourself and how that affects your relationship is one of the hardest exercises for most of my clients. We are socialized to think loving ourselves is selfish. It is viewed as egotistical and somehow corrupt. But the plain truth is you must love yourself first and foremost or you will not be physically and emotionally healthy to love others. For example, I love myself so much that I take an hour a day away from my daughters to exercise and stretch. Even though my daughters are in school and the hours after school are precious and few, I need to get my exercise in so that I am strong and balanced to be my best. When I get to exercise, I am a calm, level-headed, patient, energetic and healthy mom for my daughters. If I were to decide that I need to spend more time with them and don't have the time to exercise, then the quality of the time I spend with them would diminish.

Here is another example of how I love myself and how it affects my marriage. Because I love myself, I make good food choices and time for exercise so that when my husband and I no longer have to work and our children are grown, we can go off on hiking trips, bike trails, cruises, and other fun vacations without worries of prescriptions needing to be refilled, doctor's visits, or just

27

because we don't have the energy or quality of health to go and do those fun things.

Neither of these two examples is me being selfish or egotistical. Prioritizing my health needs benefits my entire family. One of the great benefits of being healthy is having a lean body, something I enjoy as a by-product of my love for me, not my primary goal.

Separating 'food as a source of fuel to lead an amazing life' from 'living life to eat food' is difficult. We live in a very food centered society. Dates are usually at a restaurant, celebrating occasions with friends is drinks and dinner, someone passes away we take the relatives casseroles, baseball victories are pizza parties and ice cream.

Years ago, my husband had a bad habit of ordering biscuits and fried chicken if we went to a restaurant that had them on the menu. As he was getting ready to leap head first into his junk, he would reminisce, "My dad ate this all the time."

After he ate the junk, he felt awful about his food choices and his lack of discipline. He reflected that his dad's bad eating habits were eventually his downfall, as he died from heart failure after suffering too many heart attacks. Even though the thought of eating biscuits and fried chicken gave the illusion of feeling closer to his dad who my husband greatly misses, the action of eating these foods made him feel horrible.

He realizes these junk food choices are only bringing him closer to his dad by bringing him closer to his own grave, and he is able to lovingly remember how wonderful his dad was when he smells biscuits and fried chicken. He doesn't feel the need to eat the foods that eventually led to his dad's demise.

The Unsupportive Support System

I am very blessed to have a husband and family who may raise eye brows at some of the crazy ideas I come up with, but nonetheless support me. I am shocked when I have clients who share that their significant other or mom is not supportive of a change to a healthy lifestyle. This can be a difficult obstacle, but I always tell my clients and friends that you cannot use your family's resistance as an excuse for not making your health a priority.

Recently, I had a friend tell me that she and her husband were visiting in-laws and they just couldn't eat real food or get any exercise on the trip. They had to eat the food that was provided so as not to be rude. And there was no time in their busy schedule of visiting other relatives to exercise. If your in-laws love you, then they will understand if you buy and prepare your own food. And you can complete a great workout in just four minutes! *No gimmicks*, I promise. Everyone has four minutes to spare. If your in-laws don't care much for you, then you really don't have much to lose in the first place!

All kidding aside, most people bristle when someone in their close circle tries to make a lifestyle change. Humans are natural creatures of habit, and change is uncomfortable. I can name five people, off the top of my head, whose day would be ruined if they had to take a detour route to work. And this is just a commute! I know ladies who wrote angry letters to a cosmetic company that changed the name of their favorite shade of lipstick from Renaissance Red to Romance Red. Your loved ones don't hate you for making a change, they hate the change. And if you can stick it out, it will become familiar and no longer be a change.

Sometimes you have to take the lead in change; no one said it would be an easy task. "Weird eaters", "difficult eaters", "ruining everyone's fun" "acting anorexic": I've heard all of these lines from co-workers. I am not one for peer pressure and always shrug it off. On a work trip where I refused to partake in junk food, I was told, "Just relax, we are on a semi-vacation." One of the most relaxing feelings I have ever had was after a great, exhausting work out while fasting. Eating junk food, skipping work outs and then dealing with a bloated gut, constipation and body issues does not help me relax.

Remind your loved ones that you aren't asking them to eat the foods you are choosing or to work out if they are not willing. You can offer them information and talk with them about the important changes you are making for a better, healthier you. You can communicate to them that you support and are not judging their choice not to make the changes with you and tell them you love them. I find that when you are open and honest about your feelings, no one will put you down. Confusion is the real root for resentment.

"Supportive friends" who offer you a cookie "to be nice" or tease you that "you aren't any fun" because you won't go to happy hour with them need to be reassessed. Be mindful that you are a reflection of the company you keep. Surround yourself with happy, healthy, and strong people. They will influence you to keep comparable standards. Surrounding yourself with unhappy and weak people will find you sitting around complaining about life. You may not get to choose your relatives, but you do get to choose your friends; choose wisely.

The Digestion of MyPlate

The USDA food pyramid and the new MyPlate are heavily substantiated by a mountain of scientists, government agencies and a multi-million dollar ad campaign. Why are those who follow these principles the fattest, most medication dependent on earth?

Let's examine how carbohydrates, fat and protein in the same meal are metabolized and how a carbohydrate based diet, as the MyPlate suggests, affects your health.

If you eat a carbohydrate (and all carbohydrates turn into glucose as soon as they hit your lips) and dietary fats, your body will use the carbohydrate as fuel first and store the dietary fat (think wheat bagel with cream cheese). Dietary fat in the presence of carbohydrates is metabolized very differently than dietary fat in the absence of carbohydrates.

The body must prioritize tasks, and as previously discussed, anything over five grams of glucose in the blood stream is toxic. The carbohydrates that are converted into glucose pose a higher threat than the dietary fat; the excess glucose must be stored in the muscle tissue, burned off and/or swept out of the blood stream.

A standard wheat bagel has 52 grams of carbohydrates (this information can be found on the nutrition label of every food product), and roughly four of those grams are fiber. Thus, 48 grams convert directly to glucose. Since five grams of carbohydrate are roughly the equivalent of one teaspoon (which is four grams) of glucose, 48 grams translate into 9.6 teaspoons of glucose in the blood. That is approximately 4.6 teaspoons **over** the standard safe five grams for blood glucose levels.

What's not stored in the muscle tissue is burned off as quickly as possible; forcing you to burn the glucose, not the dietary fat. Plus, your cells can only burn so much glucose at a time. The dietary fat in the cream cheese is immediately stored as fat. What happens to the rest of the carbohydrates that aren't being stored in the muscles or burned? It is converted into saturated fat, and we know where that goes…double chin, hips, and shudder…visceral fat.

When carbohydrates and protein (think eggs and toast) are eaten together glycation occurs. Glycation is a glucose and a protein molecule bound together. When this happens, insulin is unable to metabolize them properly and they become sticky, misshapen and malfunction. This leads to the degenerative aging process of tissues. The protein is damaged and unable to be used to repair cells and tissue. Over time, the glycation of proteins will damage and injure tissues and organs. If your blood is too sugary, then glycation will accelerate everywhere, from your eyes to your ankles leading to the loss of collagen in the blood and skin, Alzheimer's disease, the loss of eye sight and more.

Because blood always has glucose in it, a certain amount of glycation is always taking place throughout the body. The higher the blood glucose level, the more radical is the glycation. Under normal conditions, glycation is a very slow and steady affair. The process accelerates whenever your glucose levels are raised, but if you stay within the normal 80-90 mg/dl blood glucose limits then it doesn't accelerate.

Ingesting carbohydrates is not detrimental if you determine your personal tolerance level to carbohydrates. Not everyone's carbohydrate tolerance is the same, and through the use of a glucometer, you can define and construct a menu that fits your specific dietary needs for your optimal health. Having the ability to eat carbohydrates and seeing how those carbohydrates affect your body will result in helping you determine the timing, portion and even limiting of certain carbohydrates.

Over the past thirty years, we have been convinced that dietary fat is evil and to be hated. An example of confusion over dietary fat is cholesterol. We've been advised that if an egg contains cholesterol and we eat that egg, *our* cholesterol will raise. The problem with this logic is that the dietary cholesterol that is in food and the cholesterol that is diagnostically tested for are not the same.

Diagnostic tests for cholesterol lump cholesterol as a whole into one bucket. The cholesterol that is in an egg is essential fat that provides stability to every cell in the body. The cholesterol that is diagnostically tested for is composed of three separate lipoproteins: *High Density Lipoproteins (HDL)* is good cholesterol. HDL scavenges the blood looking for *Low Density Lipoproteins (LDL)*, the bad cholesterol. HDL scrubs the walls of blood vessels, keeping the blood vessels clean, which prevents damage. Damage to the blood vessels can lead to a hardening and narrowing of arteries, which blocks and restricts blood flow. Build-up in arteries is known as plaque and this restricts the blood flow which causes a heart attack or stroke. LDL is the culprit for the damage to the blood vessels. It accumulates and breaks down the blood vessels increasing your risk for heart disease or stroke.

Last is *Very Low Density Lipoproteins (VLDL)*. VLDL is more dangerous than LDL because it contains triglycerides. VLDL is created from alcohol, excess calories and converted sugar (glucose).

Eggs do not contain HDL, LDL or VLDL. These lipoproteins are produced by the liver during digestion. What causes high LDL and VLDL readings? A carbohydrate based diet. However, eating foods that contain cholesterol do raise your total cholesterol levels *temporarily* (during digestion).

Who benefits from diets based in carbohydrates? The food industry, diet industry, big agribusiness, and the pharmaceutical companies make a significant profit off of your carbohydrate consumption which is why the MyPlate and the prior Food Pyramids suggest 6-11 servings of whole grains a day. You do not benefit from a diet based on carbohydrates.

Media Misinformed

In my opinion, our problem with poor food choices and fat accumulation is misinformation. I think we are media misinformed and market-scammed, and it is impossible to know which diet or exercise plan to follow.

For example, how many real people do you know who have followed low calorie, mail-order processed food programs – the ones commonly seen on infomercials with fantastic claims, a celebrity spokesman and usually, a handful of really inspiring before and after photos – and gotten the health and physique levels that they desired from it? And more importantly, maintained those levels for years after?

How about the nutritional supplements out there? Many of them make astounding health claims with "medically approved" stamps of approval. But how many people do you actually know who changed their lives by drinking acai berry juice?

The marketing term for processing a food is "adding value." Highly processed foods can be made from cheaper raw materials – the quality doesn't matter if they are heavily processed - and sold for more money. Word play is a common trap consumers fall into when shopping for food or looking for an exercise routine.

For example, as I keep saying for emphasis, all carbohydrates, except for fiber, turn into glucose (sugar) in the body as soon as they hit your lips. Wouldn't it be easier for a consumer to read "Sugar" on a nutrition label versus "Total Carbohydrate, Sugars, and Fiber"? This leads the consumer to believe there is a definite difference between a carbohydrate and sugar, when there is not. It also makes it impossible to determine how much of a product is harmless fiber as opposed glucose-morphing carbohydrates.

My daughters think it is a novel idea to test their blood glucose levels. They eat something and then ask me to test them to see how it impacted them. I think it is fantastic they are taking an interest in their health already. One morning, shortly after I began my initial experiment of testing myself, my oldest daughter asked me to test her after she had a bowl of cereal. This cereal boasted being "Gluten Free" as it was made with rice. I tested her sixty minutes after she ate the cereal and her blood glucose level was 137. Needless to say, we no longer buy cereal. It would be more beneficial to eat the box the cereal comes in.

Marketers use terminology to confuse you. The latest carbohydrate confusion is net carbs. Products such as flat breads claim to be low net carb because they use alcohol sugars, non-foods that aren't completely absorbed in the blood stream and contribute less to blood glucose levels. But alcohol sugars are plain and simple chemicals.

Merchants want to sell their product to you. Selling their product makes them money. They have no interest in whether or not their product keeps you healthy. Merchants spend millions of dollars on marketing to entice and convince you to purchase their products. If a label boasts "Vegetarian Fed" and you confuse that term with "Grass Fed," then their marketing team has done their job.

What is the benefit of Grass Fed meat? It is more nutrient dense (B-vitamins, beta-carotene, vitamin E, vitamin K, and trace minerals like magnesium, calcium, and selenium.) Grass fed meat has Omega-3, the "good" naturally occurring fat. Vegetarian fed meat is livestock that was fed grains and corn. Grains and corn are vegetarian foods, yes. But corn and grain fed meat is higher in saturated fat. You are what you eat.

Another common term on labeling meat is "Free Range". Free Range means the livestock has access to walk around outside. There are no regulations denoting how long they have to be outside or the quality of their access to outside.

Another popular marketing term is "All Natural." Merchants are allowed to label their products "All Natural" even if the product contains high fructose corn syrup (HFCS). HFCS is created in a laboratory where an enzymatic processing is used to convert some of the glucose into fructose to produce a high level of sweetness. Some research has shown that HFCS leads to more and more abnormal weight gain than simple sugar. But because HFCS starts as corn it can be labeled "All Natural."

This is simply being dishonest and a marketing hype to sell, you, the consumer, a product that you feel is wholesome and suitable.

We need to educate ourselves about the foods we eat and even the foods our food is eating, or we are going to get sick and fat. We have some great doctors out there but they don't have all the answers. *You* need to be in charge of *your* health. Medication is not a cure; changing your lifestyle and eating habits is the cure. The answers to health aren't complicated. I can sum it up with eat *real* food. Eat less food. Exercise daily. Drink water. Get plenty of *good* rest. These things aren't complicated; but with marketing confusion and misinformation it can be daunting and one of the hardest tasks you take on.

You aren't lazy

Fat accumulation and hunger are symptoms of a bigger problem. As with any disease, you cannot focus on the symptom and hope the problem goes away. My clients are not lazy people. They desperately want and try to lose weight. They have tried all the diets out there and have had gym memberships most of their lives.

I have heard the most heartbreaking stories of their woes with fat. One lady shared with me that when she went anywhere, she would walk into the room and look around to see if she was fattest person there. She didn't want to be the fattest person in the room everywhere she went, but she didn't know how to cure this symptom.

It's not like we aren't trying to slim down! The fitness industry is a billion dollar operation! Americans try gym memberships and diets to no avail because the carbohydrate-glucose monster ALWAYS wins. It's not a lack of will power; you have to change your approach, an approach to turn the screams of the carbohydrate-glucose burning monster off. By switching from being a carbohydrate fuel burner to a fat burner, you will gain control of your health.

Optimal health gives you longevity, so that when you are in your 60's and 70's, and hopefully beyond, and you retire from work, you can go on cruises, and hike and bike trails across this great land. You don't want to be tied to the house or a medical care facility because of medication schedules or doctor's appointments or because you just don't feel well enough to do those things.

What you do today is providing you with your current results. If you don't have the results you want, then you have to change your approach. Our oversized appetites are because we have become a Nation of carbohydrate eaters. It's really quite a phenomenon, because sugar and/or grains (carbohydrates) using a market schemed name, are in everything! Don't believe me? On your next grocery shopping trip read the ingredient labels of any item. I bet you'll be surprised.

Sustained high blood glucose levels ruin your insulin's ability to get the correct signals to your cells to shed weight, be disease free and healthy. If you can control your blood glucose levels you will be health, disease free, and fit and trim.

Chapter Four:

The basics

The glucometer is hands down the best tool for a healthy body, and one of the many benefits of a healthy body, is a lean body. During this program, through the use of a glucometer, you will manage and understand how to sustain blood glucose levels between 80-90 mg/dl.

Your first step will be to purchase a glucometer. Glucometers are inexpensive and your standard retail stores and drugstores carry them. They range in price from free (with rebate) to around $25. It is personal preference as to which glucometer you buy and use. The test strips are the most expensive part about home glucose testing. Ranging from $1.00 each to cheaper if you buy larger quantities, and depending on your meter you can find a lower rate online.

My advice on the expense is to ask you what is more expensive: purchasing $60 worth of glucose test strips or budgeting for routine health and pharmaceutical related bills?

Do not be afraid of the pin prick to test your blood glucose levels. The required amount of blood is a tiny speck and the needle prick is barely felt. Test on the sides of your fingertip pads. Most lancets have a dial from 1-5. 1 is the lightest prick. I generally use a 2; my daughter's use a 1; and my husband, whose hands, are calloused, uses a 5. And the 5 barely breaks his skin!

Begin each day by testing your blood glucose levels upon waking and in a fasted state (prior to any food consumption) and record your level.

The other times I recommend you test, are before a meal and ninety minutes after that meal, and after you work out.

Your blood glucose level before you eat should not be over 90 mg/dl. If your levels are over 90 mg/dl, it is best not to eat and perform a twenty-minute brisk walk, or some form of aerobic exercise to allow your muscles to expend their stored glucose and absorb the excess out of your blood, so that you can obtain a glucose level of 80-90 mg/dl.

When I first started testing my blood glucose levels, I was surprised by certain foods that we think of as "health foods" that spiked my glucose levels. For example, grapes and tomatoes spiked my glucose levels into the 100's. Starch, such as potatoes and rice and treats, increases my glucose levels, but I still allow myself these foods, I just alter the timing of them or use portion control and a brisk walk after I eat.

Remember, having carbohydrates is not necessarily detrimental. However, you need to find *your* personal tolerance level to carbohydrates. **Not everyone's carbohydrate tolerance is the same** and through the use of a glucometer, you can define and construct a menu that fits your specific dietary needs for your optimal health. Having the ability to eat carbohydrates and seeing how these carbohydrates affect your body will help you determine the timing, portion and even the elimination of certain carbohydrates.

Record all your test scores. Ninety minutes postprandial (after eating) blood glucose levels should be roughly the same score as your score prior to that meal or at the very least under 90 mg/dl. If it is not, you should do some sort of aerobic activity to sweep excess glucose out of your blood and get your blood glucose level to under 90 mg/dl.

By engaging in aerobic activity to activate your muscles and assist your pancreas in returning your blood glucose levels to under 90 mg/dl, you are giving this precious organ, the pancreas, a break from having to work too hard by producing additional insulin. The more insulin your pancreas produces, the higher your risk of all those dreaded conditions and diseases and excess fat accumulation.

The test after you work out may give readings over 90 mg/dl because your body produces another hormone called, cortisol, during exercise. This is normal and good! It is an appropriate and temporary, anti-inflammatory response to the work out. Your blood glucose levels should return to less than 90 md/dl shortly after you are done.

This program is designed to help you obtain blood glucose levels between 80-90 mg/dl, not to diagnose pre-diabetes or diabetes. If you are concerned about your test scores, please make an appointment with your doctor to discuss.

Through your manipulation of a menu of real food ingredients, the timing of treats and starch, the use of fasting, and an exercise program you design for your fitness level, this book will help you to obtain glucose levels of 80-90 mg/dl which will result in a lean, healthy body.

If you continue to experience glucose levels of over 99 mg/dl you should talk with your doctor; but you should also eliminate foods that cause your glucose levels to spike, add additional exercise and add more fasts to your routine.

Journaling

The use of a glucometer will get you out of your comfort zone. You will be faced with proof that what you just ate isn't good for you, that your food choices are making you fat and unhealthy. When that happens, you can decide upon two actions. Take that food out of your diet or alter the timing of that meal/food item in your diet around exercise or a fast. Of course, you can completely ignore the results and rationalize somehow that it isn't "that bad".

Every blind spot comes at a cost. We all have comfort zones, like thermostats, and the idea that we are aware of something that can help us but don't actually make use of that knowledge, brings about a feeling of cognitive dissonance and takes us out of that comfort zone.

The quickest way back into that comfort zone is not to acknowledge that we are playing a role in hindering our own progress, but to construct an explanation that in fact, nothing of the sort is happening. You must accept that if you don't have the results that you want, it is your fault. Your health is your responsibility. Knowledge is free...so is effort.

In the pages provided, or in a separate journal, record your meals, blood glucose levels (fasting in the morning, before and after your meals, and after you exercise) and workouts. Be explicit and specific. For example when you record a meal give details about the meal preparation: was it relatively easy to prepare or difficult, how did it taste, the texture and smell? How did you feel after you ate the meal, i.e. bloated, agitated, sleepy, or energized, etc? These details help you fine tune your self-designed menu. For example, some people are more glucose tolerant of certain foods, i.e. fruit, while others are more sensitive and may need to use strict portion control or only have those foods after an exercise session – or eliminate them altogether.

Record and journal exercise, too. Include notes on whether the workout was too easy or too hard and how you felt during and after the work out: tired, energized, beat up, injured, etc. This will help you design a tailored exercise plan to your specific needs. There is never a need to do an exercise that causes you pain or you are not able to perform properly. Not everyone wants or needs to do Olympic weight lifts and some people want more than just body weight exercises. Your exercise routine should make you feel good, refreshed and empowered. You won't get it right in twenty-one days, but don't give up! I've been working out for over eighteen years and am constantly changing my routine and focus depending on my current goals (i.e. a half marathon, a mud run, an obstacle course, or dead lifting twice my body weight). The key is *to get* weight challenging exercise, not just cardio.

Journaling will show the relationship and will aid you in identifying the cause and effect of your exercise and diet in relation to your health. Journaling allows you to stop, pay attention *and* listen to yourself. There are no rules to journaling other than *doing* it! No need to worry about messiness, grammar, poor writing; it's all OK, as long as *you* understand what is recorded.

I have been journaling my life events since I was eleven-years-old. It has been an integral part of my success today. My journals are my close, intimate, accepting, trusting, caring, honest, non-judgmental, and perfect friends. My journals are the reason I am able to write this book, to help you on your journey to health, and a lean body.

Your journal gives you the opportunity to develop control and build confidence in who you are and the choices that you make about your health. You are able to shift from the recorder, to an observer or counselor, and this leads to self-discovery by clarifying thoughts, feelings and behavior. The cause and effect of events can clarify result in a change in your behavior. Journaling can help you find the missing pieces to your ultimate health.

40

The **Real** Food Rules

The fabulous meals in the menu section of this book are made with *real* food. What is *real* food? *Real* foods are foods in their most basic form. Foods made from grains are to be avoided on this program because of the inflammation they cause in the gut from the lectin they contain and the high blood glucose spike. Lectin damages the intestinal system (your gut) by binding the sugars of cells in the gut and the blood cells and initiating an inflammatory response. This inflammatory response in your gut can cause tears in the stomach lining and stomach acid leaks into the body causing a slew of problems like neurodegenerative disease, inflammatory bowel disease, infectious and autoimmune diseases. Grains include: wheat, any kind of flour, bread, pizza, tortilla, sandwiches, oats, grits, cream of wheat, cereal (all kinds), ice cream sandwiches, cookies, crackers, pasta, noodles, macaroni, couscous, cornbread, buckwheat, cracked wheat, quinoa, sorghum, millet, and amaranth.

Legumes also have lectin, but it can cook out if beans are rinsed, soaked and cooked well.

Avoid all sugar to include: sucrose, fructose, dextrose, turbanado, corn syrup, high fructose corn syrup, maltodextrin, maltose, and glucose.

All alcohol use should be in extreme moderation and if your goal is to lose weight you should not have alcohol.

Water, tea, and coffee are the only drinks.

There will be no non-foods in this program. Non-foods are sugar free foods or food made with artificial sweeteners and chemicals to include: splenda, sucralose, saccharin, aspartame, and acesulfame potassium. Basically, if you can't pronounce it, don't eat it. Another good rule of thumb is, if it doesn't rot, throw it out.

Your diet is as follows in this order: meat/fish/poultry, eggs, veggies, nuts, and then adding in fruit, potatoes and rice. A common downfall of the Paleo diet is replacing foods that had grains with fruit and nuts. Nuts are a good source of healthy fats, not protein, and the serving size is relatively small, about ¼ cups. It is too easy to over eat your healthy fats in nuts if nuts are the main staple of your diet. And there comes a point when too much dietary fat will cause fat accumulation. Remember fruit is still a carbohydrate and should be eaten as tolerated. Using a glucometer will allow you to determine exactly how much and the timing of fruit, potatoes and rice your body can tolerate.

One of the most common complaints about eating real food is the cost. I think the cost needs to be broken down into relative terms.

The first relative aspect is comparable cost. If you have comparable amounts of junk food with real food than yes, junk food is cheaper. Calorie for calorie, junk food is cheaper. However, you will require less real food then junk food as the glucose monster is switched off.

More important is the long term impact of the cost of food. The immediate gratification of saving money on your food selections today will add up with long term implications of a low quality diet. You will face frequent doctor and specialist insurance co-pays and/or medical bills, medication costs and missed days at work.

Another cost is clothes. As your waist line increases you will have to purchase bigger clothes every few years. This can be expensive if you have to wear a suit to work.

Cigarettes are very expensive but that doesn't stop smokers from purchasing them. Soda is expensive but soda addicts won't skip this purchase. The cost of quality food simply comes down to priorities.

Habit Forming

I am designing this program in a twenty-one day format. To be honest you probably won't master this in twenty-one days. But if you can dedicate twenty-one consistent days to this program, you are on your way to a lifestyle habit and can stop struggling with making healthy food choices, getting daily exercise, remembering to drink water and getting proper sleep.

You'll have a good idea of what is going on inside your body and you'll be able to keep this in mind when making food choices, choosing to stay up late to watch that television program, or choosing between getting that workout in or skipping it. Better information will provide you with better health.

Twenty-one consistent days will allow you to quiet the glucose-sugar monster screams and make food choices based on actual needs instead of cravings. After listening to your body's specific needs for twenty-one days it will be hard to go back to the ignorant bliss of bad health habits.

This program will let you *feel* what healthy is and you can recognize how eating certain foods makes you sick. You won't be tired and lethargic; your stomach won't be bloated; you will have started to lose excess weight; your skin will clear up; mysterious joint pain will go away. There will be numerous benefits to the first twenty-one days that will make it easy to decide to continue pursuing and perfecting this lifestyle.

Again, there are no gimmicks here. You will struggle during these twenty-one-days. While you don't have to give up happy hour, you do have to give up the amount of times you drink at happy hours. You can go to happy hour with your friends, and join in the conversation and fun, without drinking. You can still be social without drinking and eating.

There will be times when you are too tired to exercise, and you will have to drum up some motivation to get the work out done. Sometimes picking an easier and shorter workout when you are tired will help you get the workout in, and there is nothing saying you can't add on to it if you get revved up once you have started!

43

I encourage you to keep eating real foods, test your blood glucose levels, get exercise and find a routine that you can live with and stay healthy. Practice makes perfect and by no means will you be perfect after twenty-one days.

Time Management

I hear all the time from clients and in general conversations with people that they don't have time to exercise. I have taken the liberty of breaking down a standard time frame because managing your time is a strategic piece to being successful at health.

There are 168 hours (7x24) in the week. If 8 of those are spent (should be spent!) sleeping each night that leaves 112 (7x8 = 56. 168-56). If you work the standard 40 hours (8x5) that leaves 72 (112-40) and let's say you have to commute to work (2 hours per day 2x5 =10) that leaves you with 62 hours a week of "free time".

That's a lot of time. Now I know realistically you have about six hours a day during your work week that is yours.

How are you spending those six hours? Watching television? Playing on the internet? Gaming? Are you spending any of those six hours on personal growth? Reading? Writing? Learning? Exercising? Meal Planning?

It's time for you to focus on productive thoughts, positive energy and plans. Let go of any animosity, resentment, envy, or jealousy. These are all negative thoughts that will tear you down in a heartbeat. They can ruin a good day. Let go of it whether you are imposing these feelings on yourself or you feel these energies coming from others.

When you manage your time poorly, junk starts to pour into all aspects of your life, not just your diet. Spending those free six free hours in the form of television, video games, and internet surfing is mind junk, just like a donut is junk to your diet.

How you spend your time comes down to your priorities. If your health is a priority you will spend some of your free time planning your meals, getting exercise, reading, writing and further educating yourself.

It is time to establish a time management plan. Ask yourself are you spending any of your free six hours exercising? I would love for everyone who reads this book to take away a new healthier lifestyle, but if you the only take one thing away from this book, I hope it is that you can work out in *your own home*, with minimal or no equipment in twelve minutes.

Are you spending any of these six hours planning your meals? Again you have to prepare to be successful. It is JUST AS EASY A CHOICE TO BUY/PREPARE REAL FOOD AS IT IS TO BUY JUNK FOOD.

Let's start turning the junk off and empower your mind with positive things that will enable you to grow in a positive direction.

Take advantage of the journaling aspect of this program, and plan your day. Include your commute, any meetings, doctor's appointment, extracurricular activities, running the pet to the vet, grocery store trips, meal prep, your exercise time, even time with your spouse.

Putting your thoughts down on paper is a good way to organize them, and it's a great way to see that everything you need to get done in a day may just not get done. This will prevent you from stressing about your to-do list and prioritize what needs to get done and what can wait for another day.

Priorities.....what are you going to do with your six hours today?

Chapter Five:

Exercise....

Yes, you have to

Exercise is a great tool to help keep your blood glucose levels at the desired 80-90 mg/dl. When you exercise, your muscles are depleted and to restore their energy they suck excess glucose out of your blood stream; not to mention that when you exercise, you create more muscle tissue. Muscle is a storage depot for glucose. If when you exercise you are creating more muscle tissue, then obviously you will have more room for glucose to be sucked up out of your blood. Your muscle tissue is where glucose *should* be, *not* floating around your blood causing your pancreas to work overtime or being converted into fat because there is nothing else for your body to do with it.

A super-efficient exercise at sucking glucose out of the blood stream is High Intensity Interval Training otherwise known as HIIT. HIIT is all about intensity. To perform HIIT, first properly warm up for about two minutes of the exercise to be performed at a much slower pace. Then you spend six to twelve minutes going back and forth between a 20-30 second intense pace of that exercise and a 20-30 second (matching) rest. A great example of HIIT is doing sprints. Sprint as fast as you can for 30 seconds, then walk for 30 seconds, and repeat for six to twelve repetitions. The short burst of intensity empties the muscle of energy (glucose). To restore their depleted energy, the muscle will suck glucose out of the blood, causing blood glucose levels to decrease. The pancreas doesn't have to work as hard.

And for the love of your health, do not be afraid to lift heavy weights. Lifting heavy weights doesn't make you bulky. Having too much body fat makes you bulky. You can see full body pictures of me throughout this book, I weigh approximately 136 pounds. I currently Dead Lift 240#s, Back Squat 235#, Front Squat 155#, and can Clean and Press 130#. I am not bulky, nor do I look like a man. It's not easy to put on muscle mass; you will not look like a muscle bound steroid freak from any of the advice in this book.

Stress

When you are exposed to a stressful situation, your adrenal glands pump out stress hormones to prepare your body to cope with the situation and for eminent extreme exertion like running from a bear! Your heart starts to pump harder, your blood pressure rises, your blood's ability to clot becomes easier (just in case that bear gets you and you are wounded), and your blood flow is directed to the digestive system to help make fuel for the escape. This function is the hormone called cortisol. Cortisol raises your blood glucose levels and this is a normal process if your body is in a stressful situation (working out, being chased, etc). After the tense situation, your cells will resume to their normal functions. But when you are fighting chronic stress, you stay in this over heightened metabolic stage of distress.

This is not good for several reasons. It increases your risk of stroke from the clotting measures and higher blood pressure. It can cause a heart attack because your heart is working harder, and it can cause diabetes as your blood glucose levels are constantly high. Fat will start to accumulate all over your body, especially in your waist (remember that visceral fat) compounding the problem.

When you are stressed, you are constantly in the "fight-or-flight," turbo-charged mode, and your body undergoes more and more wear and tear. You will quickly wear out, age, become diseased, and die. This is too much wear and tear on your body.

Cortisol gets a bad reputation because of our continued high levels of stress. Too much cortisol can suppress the immune system by "muting" the white blood cells. Cortisol counter acts with insulin causing your blood glucose levels to be continually high, and will reflect in your body by causing weight gain and loss of skin collagen making you look older quicker. 'Quit stressing, it's giving you wrinkles' is true! Too much cortisol will damage short term memory ability because cortisol attacks cells in the hippocampus that are responsible for short term memory, and weaken the immune system by weakening the anti-inflammatory response.

Finding the right balance of cortisol is a very complex art.

47

Supplements

I frequently get asked my thoughts on supplements. Plain and simple, save your money. Supplements should not be the cornerstone of your diet. There are a few that I use. However they aren't magic.

Niacin. This is the best pre-workout supplement out there, because if you take a 500mg Niacin and don't get moving, you are going to be very uncomfortable very fast. Your skin will flush; flushing is red and itchy skin. This is completely normal. The less you move, the harder you flush.

Don't waste your money on the more expensive flush-free Niacin, it is not the same, and it doesn't work. Plain Niacin is cheap. If you have never taken Niacin before I recommend starting with 250 mg. Then progress up to 500mg.

Niacin opens up all the capillaries in your body and lets the blood flow better; basically you warm up faster. Other benefits of niacin are stabilizing blood sugar levels and increasing HDL.

Probiotics. Buy in the powder form and one that requires refrigeration. Gut health is essential to health. Probitoics should be taken on an empty stomach for effectiveness.

Let's talk poop! I know shhhhhh - don't say that publicly, right?! No one ever wants to talk poop but it is important.

First things first, frequency - how often should you go? Every day, period. If you eat every day you should poop every day although it takes about three days for what you eat to complete the digestion process (I'm sure you ate three days ago).

How about color? It should be brown, the brown color comes from bile (good job probiotics!) from the liver; this is an indication that your liver is functioning properly. Black could mean excessive vitamins or internal bleeding (colon cancer); grey could mean your liver is not working properly. Get those symptoms checked out by a doctor.

Smell - oh man it should STINK! Why? Because your gut has (should have) tons of bacteria and bacteria (go probiotics!) help with digestion and the metabolic process. So be proud of your stink! It means you are healthy. I don't suggest you come out of a public stall and do a suck it hand gesture to those gagging at the sink...but a smug smile is acceptable.

How do you get brown stinky poop every day? Lots of water, exercise and eating real food. Happy pooping!

Magnesium aspartate – Magnesium deficiency can cause lots of problems including muscle soreness, muscle cramps, and impaired contraction of the smooth muscle tissue. Basically if you work out and you feel like you are getting extremely sore after the workout or you are getting Charlie horses, you need some magnesium. Take the recommended dosage; you will know if you have taken too much (your colon is a muscle too!)

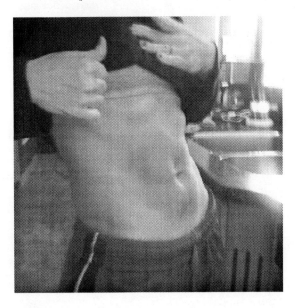

Iodine – Why iodine? Cause goiters aren't cool. On a serious note, America has become salt-phobic, and iodine deficiency is on the rise. I buy Lugol's liquid Iodine and draw a circle on my stomach and let my skin absorb it. Iodine is needed for proper function of the thyroid.

Angela

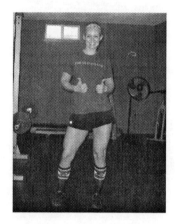

I have come to an understanding with my glucose testing. Because I am not diabetic, I do not test every day. For six months, I monitored my glucose levels when I first woke up (fasting), before and 90 minutes after a meal and after a workout. I studied the trends of what foods and other outside factors would spike my blood glucose levels to undesirable ranges.

I found I can only have sweets or red potato dishes (I don't care for rice much) in my morning meal and after I have worked out. Not necessarily as a post workout meal, but those dishes have to be eaten soon after I work out.

My fasting glucose level is higher on days when my sleep is broken or insufficient. I discovered that massages, stretching, twenty minute power naps and walking after meals all reduce my blood glucose levels.

And I incorporate a one, 24-hour fasting every other week. This fast allows my body to focus on repair instead of digestion. Digestion requires a lot of energy from your body. I believe your digestive system should get a day of rest too!

If you have a Facebook account you can like my "The Gym Cellar" page. I frequently post videos and pictures of my workouts, new recipes, motivation, invites for challenges and I debunk popular "fake" science on nutrition in a spunky, yet tart tone.

I am transparent, accessible and real. I am not a TV celebrity, a celebrity trainer, and I am not getting rich off selling products to others. I am a fitness coach. I'll be honest with you coaching is a hard, hard job. Anyone who thinks it is easy has never done it or doesn't do it correctly.

There are nights after my clients are gone, I sit in my basement gym and look around and have to gather myself before I can go upstairs to my family. I get emotionally wiped out. If a client comes in and is upset, it is my job to lift his or her spirits and get them focused on our task at hand. If they come in and don't want to get out of their comfort zone, it is my job to pull them kicking and screaming out of it to make progress and not waste their hard earned cash paying me. If they have questions I need to have the answers or find and research the answer. It's HARD work that I absolutely love.

I want you to stop thinking you are indoctrinated to fail at getting healthy and lean when you should win. And you can! The program's goal is to have *you* prioritize *your* health. Will it work? That is a question only *you* can answer. Your time is the most valuable thing you have. I ask you to give me a ***concentrated effort*** for three weeks to see the difference; a 100 percent dedication and devotion to the program. The effectiveness of this program, *if you dedicate yourself to it,* is so absolute, it could be three weeks that will change the quality of your life.

Chapter Six:

Let's Begin!

Saturday, Day One

Plan your meals for the week. Write a grocery list, you can simply highlight what you will need off of the "grocery list cheat sheet" provided. Now go groceries shopping!

Sunday, Day Two

Today should be your cooking day. To prepare for success you must plan it! Determine what you will have each day for lunch and cook up enough of that meat, i.e. barbeque up some burgers and then each day through the week you can throw one of your already cooked burgers and a veggie into a container and be on your way to work with little effort. This meat will be your lunch each day and if by chance you cannot make dinner one or two nights due to time constraints then you can eat this as well.

Use your evenings to try a new recipe. Or you can keep it simple and cook up two separate meats today, i.e. burgers and chicken breasts and use them as the base for both lunch and dinner if you know you won't have the time to cook through the week.

The meals in the recipe section can be doubled, tripled, etc. to make enough of that meal for a week. Just make sure that whatever you decide will be your base won't get soggy, hard, tough, etc. or basically unpalatable, less then desired and leaves you looking for something else. *Real* food tastes great if you put the effort into preparing it.

Having all your meat cooked and ready to re-heat leaves you no excuses – this is a very important step in making your health a priority…preparing!

Monday, Day One

Don't quit before you start!

Fasting Blood Glucose Test: _____

Meal 1: Choose a breakfast from the recipe section or a grain and sugar free meal!

90 minutes post-meal Blood Glucose Test: _____

Challenge: Week One, Day One workout and pick a visible spot for your reflection board (over your desk, fridge, bathroom mirror; anywhere you frequent often in the day).

Post Workout Blood Glucose Test: _____

Pre-meal Blood Glucose Test: _____

Meal 2: Your prepared meal

90 minutes post-meal Blood Glucose Test: _____

Pre-meal Blood Glucose Test: _____

Meal 3: Choose a dinner recipe from the recipe section or a grain and sugar free meal!

90 minutes post-meal Blood Glucose Test: _____

Tuesday, Day Two

There is a difference between interest and commitment. When you are interested in doing something, you do it when it is convenient. When you are committed you accept no excuses, only results!

Fasting Blood Glucose Test: _____

Meal 1: Choose a breakfast from the recipe section or a grain and sugar free meal!

90 minutes post-meal Blood Glucose Test: _____

Challenge: Week One, Day Two workout. Tell one person in your life that *you* love *you* and how that positively affects your relationship together.

Post Workout Blood Glucose Test: _____

Pre-meal Blood Glucose Test: _____

Meal 2: Your prepared meal.

90 minutes post-meal Blood Glucose Test: _____

Pre-meal Blood Glucose Test: _____

Meal 3: Choose a dinner recipe from the recipe section or a grain and sugar free meal!

90 minutes post-meal Blood Glucose Test: _____

Wednesday, Day Three

It matters most when no one's watching!

Fasting Blood Glucose Test: _____

Meal 1: Choose a breakfast from the recipe section or a grain and sugar free meal!

90 minutes post-meal Blood Glucose Test: _____

Challenge: Week One, Day Three workout. One hour of television today. Limit the junk.

Post Workout Blood Glucose Test: _____

Pre-meal Blood Glucose Test _____

Meal 2: Your prepared meal.

90 minutes post-meal Blood Glucose Test: _____

Pre-meal Blood Glucose Test: _____

Meal 3: Choose a dinner recipe from the recipe section or a grain and sugar free meal!

90 minutes post-meal Blood Glucose Test: _____

Thursday, Day Four

Lead by example, be a positive role model.

Fasting Blood Glucose Test: _____

Meal 1: Choose a breakfast from the recipe section or a grain and sugar free meal!

90 minutes post-meal Blood Glucose Test: _____

Challenge: Week One, Day Four workout. Kitchen push-ups! Every time you go into your kitchen today do five push-ups in addition to the daily workout.

Post Workout Blood Glucose Test: _____

Pre-meal Blood Glucose Test: _____

Meal 2: Your prepared meal.

90 minutes post-meal Blood Glucose Test: _____

Pre-meal Blood Glucose Test: _____

Meal 3: Choose a dinner recipe from the recipe section or a grain and sugar free meal!

90 minutes post-meal Blood Glucose Test: _____

Friday, Day Five

Strength and Power make everything in life easier!

Fasting Blood Glucose Test: _____

Meal 1: Choose a breakfast from the recipe section or a grain and sugar free meal!

90 minutes post-meal Blood Glucose Test: _____

Challenge: Week One, Day Five workout. On a piece of paper write down three things you are proud of yourself for. Add this to your reflection board.

Post Workout Blood Glucose Test: _____

Pre-meal Blood Glucose Test. _____

Meal 2: Your prepared meal.

90 minutes post-meal Blood Glucose Test: _____

Pre-meal Blood Glucose Test: _____

Meal 3: Choose a dinner recipe from the recipe section or a grain and sugar free meal!

90 minutes post-meal Blood Glucose Test: _____

Saturday, Day Six

Prepare for success!

Fasting Blood Glucose Test: _____

Meal 1: Choose a breakfast from the recipe section or a grain and sugar free meal!

90 minutes post-meal Blood Glucose Test: _____

Challenge: Week One, Day Six workout. Review your week's blood glucose level test results. Try eliminating the offending foods or moving the foods to post workout times to prevent the glucose spike. Use this information to prepare a grocery list and go shopping! Look through the recipe section and decide what you will need to make those meals.

Post Workout Blood Glucose Test: _____

Pre-meal Blood Glucose Test _____

Meal 2: Your prepared meal.

90 minutes post-meal Blood Glucose Test: _____

Pre-meal Blood Glucose Test: _____

Meal 3: Choose a dinner recipe from the recipe section or a grain and sugar free meal!

90 minutes post-meal Blood Glucose Test: _____

Sunday, Day Seven

Prepared people are successful people.

Fasting Blood Glucose Test: _____

Meal 1: Choose a breakfast from the recipe section or a grain and sugar free meal!

90 minutes post-meal Blood Glucose Test: _____

Challenge: Week One, Day Seven workout. Cook your meals for the week!!

Post Workout Blood Glucose Test: _____

Pre-meal Blood Glucose Test _____

Meal 2: Your prepared meal.

90 minutes post-meal Blood Glucose Test: _____

Pre-meal Blood Glucose Test: _____

Meal 3: Choose a dinner recipe from the recipe section or a grain and sugar free meal!

90 minutes post-meal Blood Glucose Test: _____

Monday, Day Eight

How strong should you be? As strong as you can get!

Fasting Blood Glucose Test: _____

Meal 1: Choose a breakfast from the recipe section or a grain and sugar free meal!

90 minutes post-meal Blood Glucose Test: _____

Challenge: Week Two, Day One workout. One hour of television today. Limit the junk.

Post Workout Blood Glucose Test: _____

Pre-meal Blood Glucose Test. _____

Meal 2: Your prepared meal.

90 minutes post-meal Blood Glucose Test: _____

Pre-meal Blood Glucose Test: _____

Meal 3: Choose a dinner recipe from the recipe section or a grain and sugar free meal!

90 minutes post-meal Blood Glucose Test: _____

Tuesday, Day Nine

Don't stomp on someone's shoulders to lift yourself up; but more importantly don't let anyone stomp on yours!

Fasting Blood Glucose Test: _____

Meal 1: Choose a breakfast from the recipe section or a grain and sugar free meal!

90 minutes post-meal Blood Glucose Test: _____

Challenge: Week Two, Day Two. Kitchen Push-ups!! Five push-ups each time you go into the kitchen in addition to the workout for the day.

Post Workout Blood Glucose Test: _____

Pre-meal Blood Glucose Test _____

Meal 2:

90 minutes post-meal Blood Glucose Test: _____

Pre-meal Blood Glucose Test: _____

Meal 3: Choose a dinner recipe from the recipe section or a grain and sugar free meal!

90 minutes post-meal Blood Glucose Test: _____

Wednesday, Day 10

Priorities; what are yours today?

Fasting Blood Glucose Test: _____

Meal 1: Choose a breakfast from the recipe section or a grain and sugar free meal!

90 minutes post-meal Blood Glucose Test: _____

Challenge: Week Two, Day Three workout. Tell another person in your life that you love yourself and how that positively affects your relationship with them.

Post Workout Blood Glucose Test: _____

Pre-meal Blood Glucose Test _____

Meal 2: Your prepared meal.

90 minutes post-meal Blood Glucose Test: _____

Pre-meal Blood Glucose Test: _____

Meal 3: Choose a dinner recipe from the recipe section or a grain and sugar free meal!

90 minutes post-meal Blood Glucose Test: _____

Thursday, Day 11

The greatest battle you will ever undertake is with yourself. Are you going to be your own worst enemy today?

Fasting Blood Glucose Test: _____

Meal 1: Choose a breakfast from the recipe section or a grain and sugar free meal!

90 minutes post-meal Blood Glucose Test: _____

Challenge: Week Two, Day Four workout. Complete a 16 hour fast into Friday. You will stop eating at 8:00 tonight and your first meal tomorrow will be at noon. You can have as much coffee, tea and water. You can also add heavy whipping cream to your coffee; however be liberal with the cream, this is about adding a bit of cream to your coffee not cheating the fast.

Post Workout Blood Glucose Test: _____

Pre-meal Blood Glucose Test. _____

Meal 2: Your prepared meal.

90 minutes post-meal Blood Glucose Test: _____

Pre-meal Blood Glucose Test: _____

Meal 3: *Eat this meal before 8 PM or skip it!* Choose a dinner recipe from the recipe section or a grain and sugar free meal!

90 minutes post-meal Blood Glucose Test: _____

Friday, Day 12

You will not succeed unless you face and overcome difficulties and prepare to accept responsibility.

Meal 1: Not until NOON. Your prepared meal.

Challenge: Week Two, Day Five workout.

Post Workout Blood Glucose Test: _____

Pre-meal Blood Glucose Test: _____

Meal 2: Choose a dinner recipe from the section or a grain and sugar free meal!

90 minutes post-meal Blood Glucose Test: _____

Saturday, Day 13

Smile. You woke up today.

Fasting Blood Glucose Test: _____

Meal 1: Choose a breakfast from the recipe section or a grain and sugar free meal!

90 minutes post-meal Blood Glucose Test: _____

Challenge: Week Two, Day Six workout. Take a look at your last two weeks blood glucose level test results. Decide what foods are causing you to spike and don't have them this week and see if that helps you maintain the 80-90 mg/dl level. Use this information to develop your grocery shopping list. Grocery Shopping!!

Post Workout Blood Glucose Test: _____

Pre-meal Blood Glucose Test _____

Meal 2: Your prepared meal.

90 minutes post-meal Blood Glucose Test: _____

Pre-meal Blood Glucose Test: _____

Meal 3: Choose a dinner recipe from the recipe section or a grain and sugar free meal!

90 minutes post-meal Blood Glucose Test: _____

Sunday, Day 14

Pain is temporary. Regret is forever. Keep going!

Fasting Blood Glucose Test: _____

Meal 1: Choose a breakfast from the recipe section or a grain and sugar free meal!

90 minutes post-meal Blood Glucose Test: _____

Challenge: Week Two, Day Seven workout. Cook your meals for the week

Post Workout Blood Glucose Test: _____

Pre-meal Blood Glucose Test _____

Meal 2: Your prepared meal.

90 minutes post-meal Blood Glucose Test: _____

Pre-meal Blood Glucose Test: _____

Meal 3: Choose a dinner recipe from the recipe section or a grain and sugar free meal!

90 minutes post-meal Blood Glucose Test: _____

Monday, Day 15

Your worst workout is the one you skip!

Fasting Blood Glucose Test: _____

Meal 1: Choose a breakfast from the recipe section or a grain and sugar free meal!

90 minutes post-meal Blood Glucose Test: _____

Challenge: Week Three, Day One workout. Write yourself a love letter. Tell yourself why you love you. Be specific and use specific examples of things you do that are awesome. Read the letter out loud to yourself in front of a mirror.

Post Workout Blood Glucose Test: _____

Pre-meal Blood Glucose Test _____

Meal 2: Your prepared meal.

90 minutes post-meal Blood Glucose Test: _____

Pre-meal Blood Glucose Test: _____

Meal 3: Choose a dinner recipe from the recipe section or a grain and sugar free meal!

90 minutes post-meal Blood Glucose Test: _____

Tuesday, Day 16

Stand for something or fall for everything.

Fasting Blood Glucose Test: _____

Meal 1: Choose a breakfast from the recipe section or a grain and sugar free meal!

90 minutes post-meal Blood Glucose Test: _____

Challenge: Week Three, Day Two workout. Add your letter to your reflection board and in addition to your workout take a 10 minute reflection walk.

Post Workout Blood Glucose Test: _____

Pre-meal Blood Glucose Test _____

Meal 2: Your prepared meal.

90 minutes post-meal Blood Glucose Test: _____

Pre-meal Blood Glucose Test: _____

Meal 3: Choose a dinner recipe from the recipe section or a grain and sugar free meal!

90 minutes post-meal Blood Glucose Test: _____

Wednesday, Day 17

The good stuff in life is hard to achieve; the bad stuff is effortless.

Fasting Blood Glucose Test: _____

Meal 1: Choose a breakfast from the recipe section or a grain and sugar free meal!

90 minutes post-meal Blood Glucose Test: _____

Challenge: Week Three, Day Three workout. One hour of television today. Limit the junk!

Post Workout Blood Glucose Test: _____

Pre-meal Blood Glucose Test. _____

Meal 2: Your prepared meal.

90 minutes post-meal Blood Glucose Test: _____

Pre-meal Blood Glucose Test: _____

Meal 3: Choose a dinner recipe from the recipe section or a grain and sugar free meal!

90 minutes post-meal Blood Glucose Test: _____

Thursday, Day 18

"Confidence is contagious. So is lack of confidence." Vince Lombardi

Fasting Blood Glucose Test: _____

Meal 1: Choose a breakfast from the recipe section or a grain and sugar free meal!

90 minutes post-meal Blood Glucose Test: _____

Challenge: Week Three, Day Four workout. A 20-hour fast! You will start this fast at 4:00 PM today and your first meal tomorrow will be at noon.

Post Workout Blood Glucose Test: _____

Pre-meal Blood Glucose Test: _____

Meal 2: Your prepared meal.

90 minutes post-meal Blood Glucose Test: _____

4:00: FAST. You can do this; mind over matter! Lots of water, tea and coffee; stay hydrated.

Friday, Day 19

Stay strong all the way to the finish line!

Fasting Blood Glucose Test: _____

Meal 1: NOON. Your prepared meal.

90 minutes post-meal Blood Glucose Test: _____

Challenge: Week Three, Day Five workout. Write down everything you own, all the material things you've purchased, i.e. car, home, clothes, jewelry, etc. If you subtract all the stuff you have accumulated are you happy with the person left? Spend some good quality time with someone you love today. No cell phones, no television or video games, no internet. Just you and them; you can play a board game, go on a walk, talk and listen to each other.

Post Workout Blood Glucose Test: _____

Pre-meal Blood Glucose Test. _____

Meal 2: Choose a recipe from the dinner section or a grain and sugar free meal.

90 minutes post-meal Blood Glucose Test: _____

<u>**Saturday, Day 20**</u>

Enthusiasm is everything.

Learning about what you are made of is always time well spent.

Fasting Blood Glucose Test: _____

Meal 1: Choose a breakfast from the recipe section or a grain and sugar free meal!

90 minutes post-meal Blood Glucose Test: _____

Challenge: Week Three, Day Six workout. Review this week's blood glucose level results. Try eliminating the offending food from your diet or moving those foods to times around exercise from that spiked your glucose levels. Make your grocery list and go shopping!

Post Workout Blood Glucose Test: _____

Pre-meal Blood Glucose Test _____

Meal 2: Your prepared meal.

90 minutes post-meal Blood Glucose Test: _____

Pre-meal Blood Glucose Test: _____

Meal 3: Choose a dinner recipe from the recipe section or a grain and sugar free meal!

90 minutes post meal Blood Glucose Test: _____

Sunday, Day 21

Live a life of substance. Wake up, go to work, eat, help kids with homework, eat, watch TV, go to bed. Do it all over again. That is NOT substance. You get ONE chance. Live a life of substance.

Fasting Blood Glucose Test: _____

Meal 1: Choose a breakfast from the recipe section or a grain and sugar free meal!

90 minutes post-meal Blood Glucose Test: _____

Challenge: Week Three, Day Seven workout. Cook your meals for the week.

Post Workout Blood Glucose Test: _____

Pre-meal Blood Glucose Test _____

Meal 2: Your prepared meal.

90 minutes post-meal Blood Glucose Test: _____

Pre-meal Blood Glucose Test: _____

Meal 3: Choose a dinner recipe from the recipe section or a grain and sugar free meal!

Mobility

Before beginning a workout plan, I highly recommend you take this simple mobility test to see how flexible your joints are. Have someone take your picture so that you can accurately assess your posture.

Having flexibility and correct mobility in your hip flexors, shoulders, wrists and ankles is the key to injury prevention. Mobility work is highly underrated, underutilized, and underappreciated. When your exercise program lacks mobility and stretching you put yourself at risk for a variety of injuries. When you are injured you can't train, but more importantly, injuries hurt.

Another key to taking good care of your muscles is soft tissue work and massage. Massages can be expensive, but adding a massage at least once a month is extremely beneficial.

Hip, ankle and spine flexibility

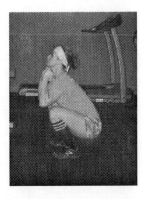

You should be able to properly squat. If you cannot squat as pictured you need to add in ankle and hip mobility work that is included in the Stretching section of this book.

Shoulder flexibility

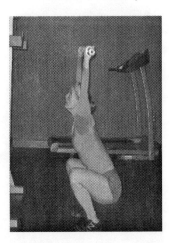

If your shoulders cannot perform the above exercise as shown you need to add in the shoulder mobility work that is in the Stretching section of this book.

Exercises

Squats

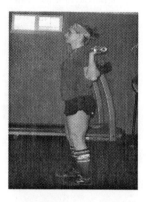

Back Squat starting position

SQUAT – **For all squats.** Feet are shoulder width apart. You will drive down THROUGH your HEELS and you will drive UP through your HEELS. NOT on your toes. Your shoulders are over your hips and you DO NOT lean forward…..THROUGH THE HEELS!

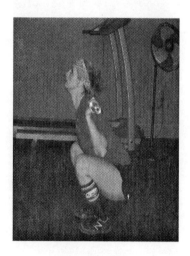

Back Squat

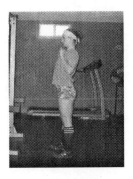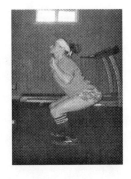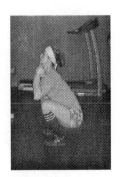

Body Weight Squat

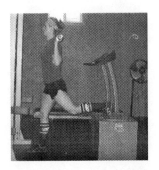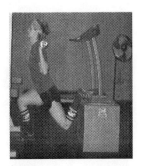

Bulgarian Squat

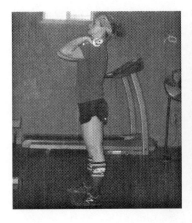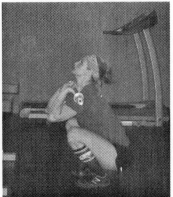

Front Squat

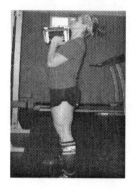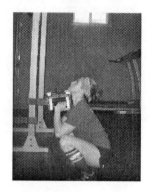

Goblet Squat

<u>Lunges</u>

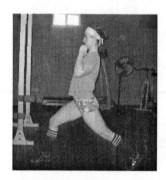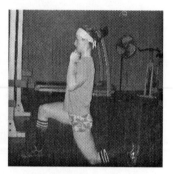

Shoulders over hips and knees don't track past your toes. The back knee goes down all the way to the knee touching the deck.

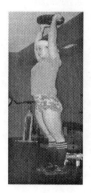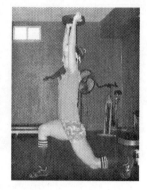

Waiter lunge

Dead Lifts

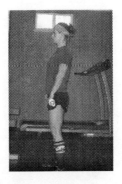

Starting position for all deadlifts, chest stays UP, shoulders BACK!

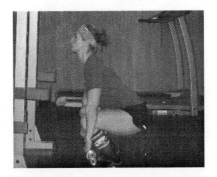

Traditional Deadlift (bar stays close to the body, scraping shins is good!)

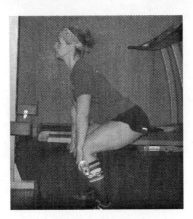

Romanian Deadlift

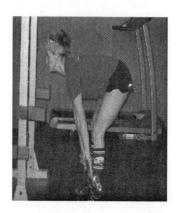

Stiff Leg Deadlift (knees bent slightly/chest up/shoulders back bar stays close to the body)

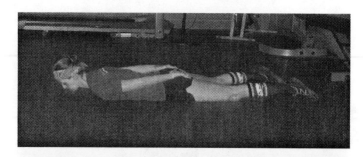

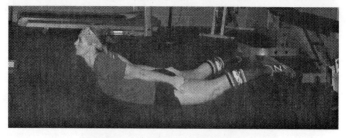

Hyper Extension (lay on belly, lift shoulders and thighs off deck. Hold for a second and release)

Boulder Shoulders

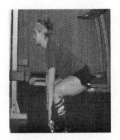

Clean & Press Start

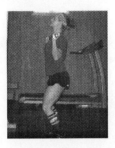

Clean & Press mid-movement

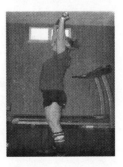

Clean and Press finish

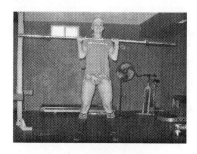

Rocky Press start

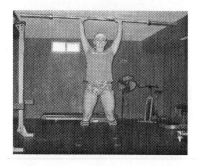

Rocky Press mid-movement

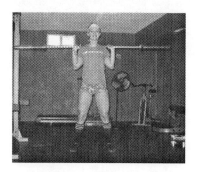

Rocky Presses finish

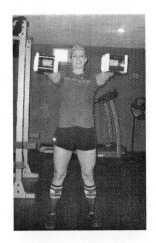

Front Lateral Raise

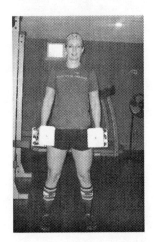

Front and Side Lateral Raise Starting position

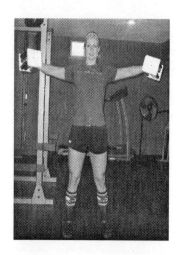

Side Lateral Raise

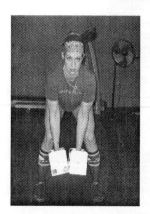 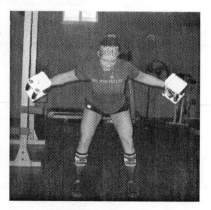

Rear Deltoid Fly

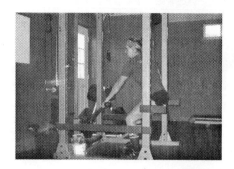 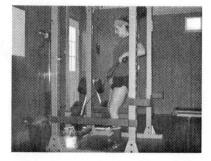

Lawn Mower Pulls

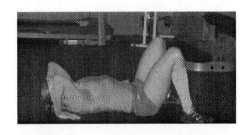

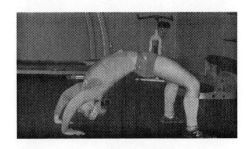

Bridges

<u>**Push-UPS!!**</u>

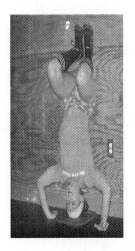 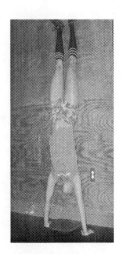

Hand Stand Push-up

Explosive push-up

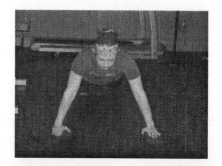

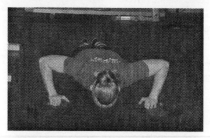

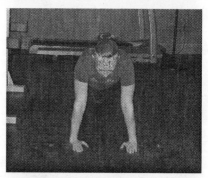

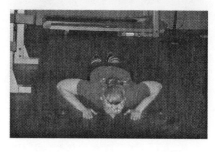

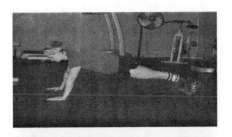

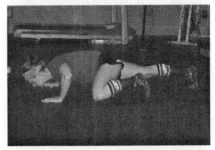

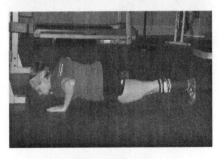

Parkour Push-up

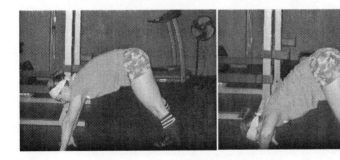

Pike Push-Up

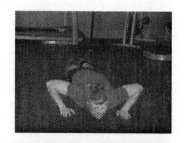

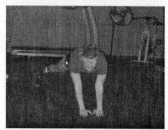

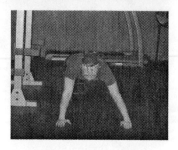

Traveling Push-up

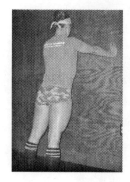 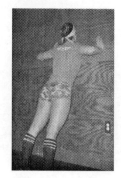

Wall Push-Up

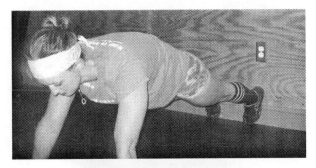

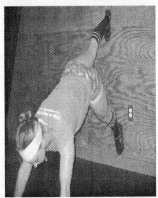

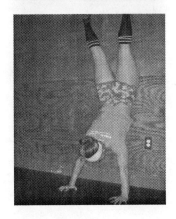

Wall Crawl

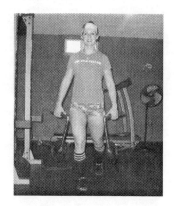

Farmer's Walk

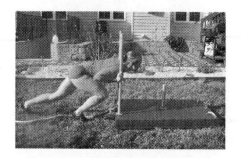

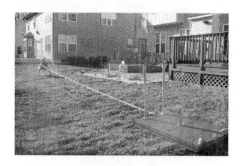

Sled Push and Sled Pulls

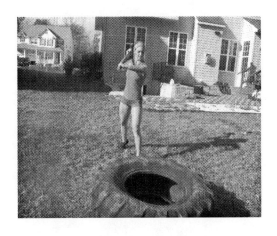

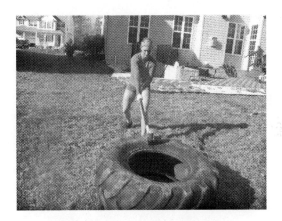

Sledge Hammer – Can be purchased at any home improvement store and vary in weight sizes.

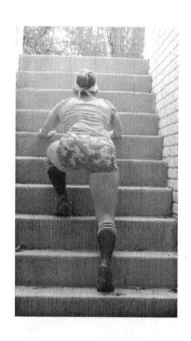

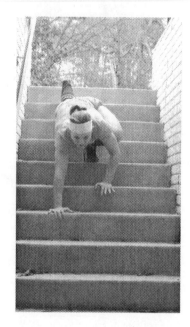

Step hand climbs up/down

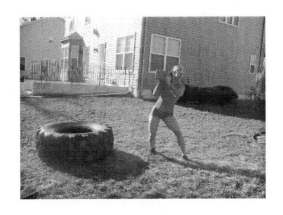

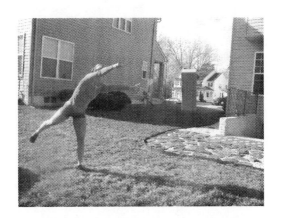

Stone Throw

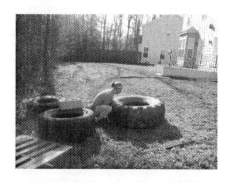

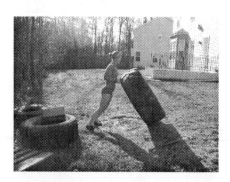

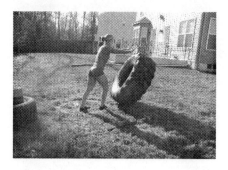

Tire flip – Keep your butt down! You can obtain a tire at any local repair shop. Garages have to pay to dispose of old tires; they will gladly give you a few for free.

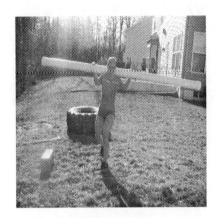

Yoke Walk

Triceps Fun

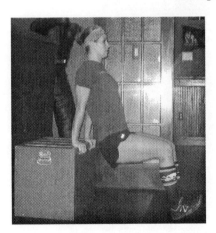 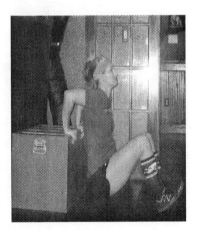

Dips

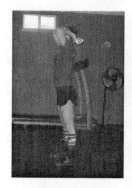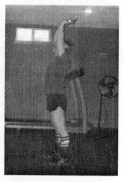

French Press

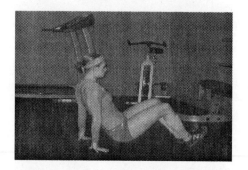

Scoot Start

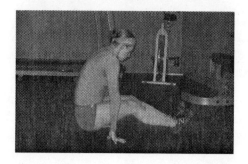

Scoot mid-position

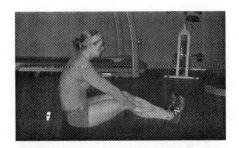

Scoot finish

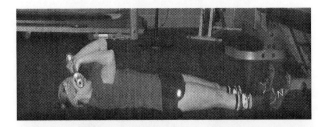

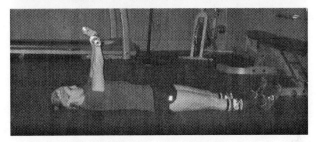

Skull Crusher

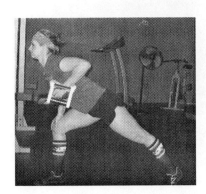 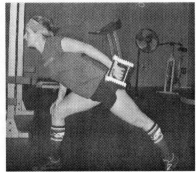

Triceps Kickback

97

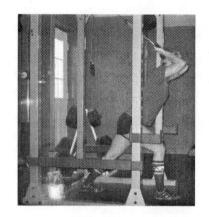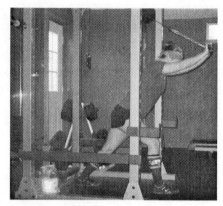

Triceps Extension

<u>Biceps</u>

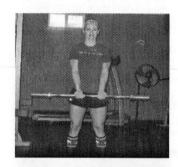

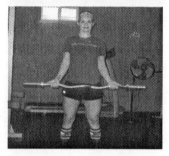

Inside Grip/Outside Grip for Barbell Curls

Pull-up/Chin-up/Mixed Grip

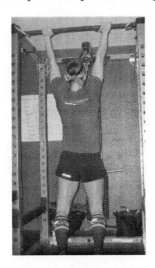

Pull-up

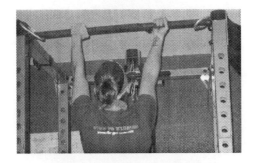

Switched Grip Pull-up

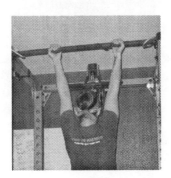

Chin-up

Jump-Jump!!

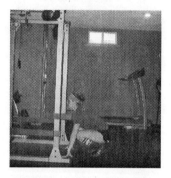

Chirpee: Jump up in the air, then crouch down, kick legs back into a push-up position, push-up, jump back into the crouch position and jump up on the pull-up bar and do a pull-up, jump down into crouched position

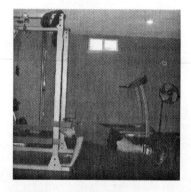

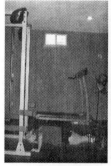 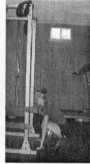 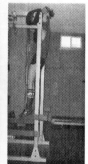

Chirpee

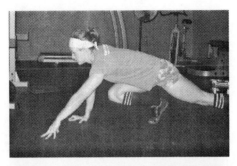

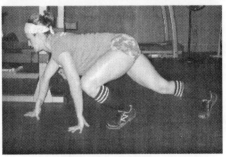

Bear Crawl

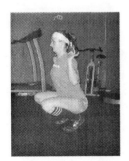 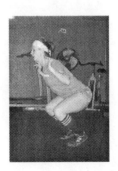 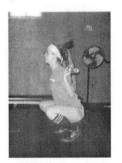

Bunny hops

Last picture is shown with weight.

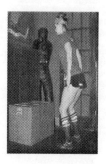

Box Jump Start

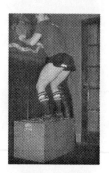

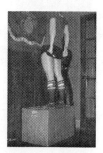

Box Jump finish (with full hip thrust)

Burpee: Jump up in the air, crouch down, kick legs back into the push-up position, push-up, jump legs back into crouch position and jump up into the air

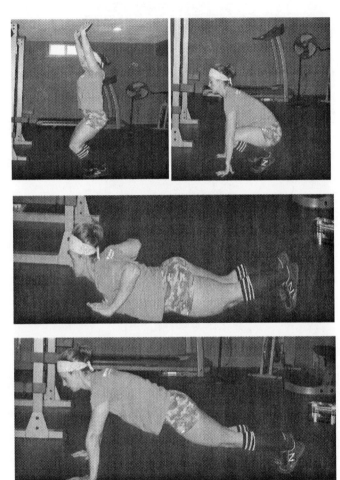

BURPEES

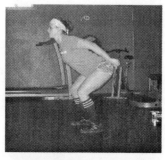

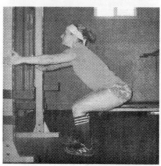

Jumps

Big leaps with both feet

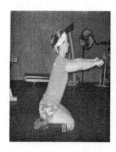 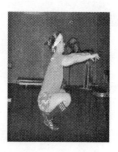 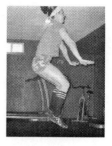

Spring Jumps

Start sitting on shins/jump up to feet or walk one knee up at a time to feet/jump in the air and pull knees to chest

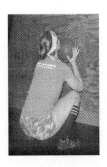

Wall Ball Starting position

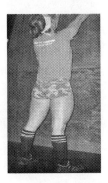

Wall ball

<u>**Ab-mazing!!**</u>

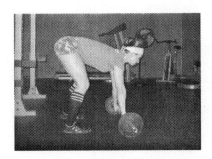 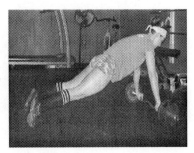

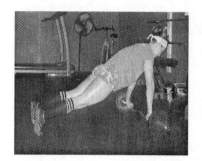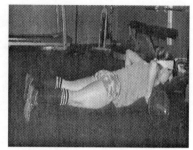

Abs Roll out

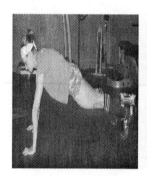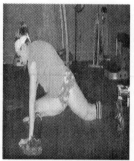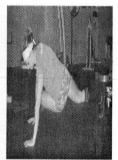

Plank Get Outs

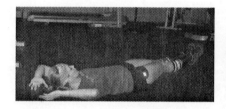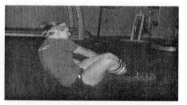

Shrimp (come up to both sides)

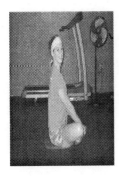 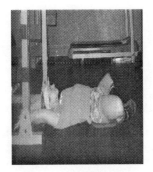 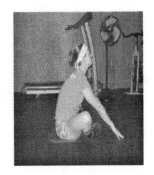

Sit-ups

(My sit-ups are done with your legs in a butterfly. You lay flat back slap the top of the floor and sit-up and slap the floor at your feet. Your legs stay in the open butterfly – this prevents you from using your thighs)

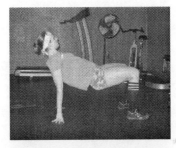

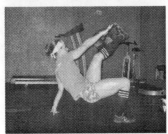

Spider kicks

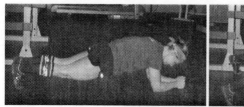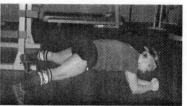

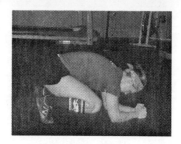

Sprawl In/Outs

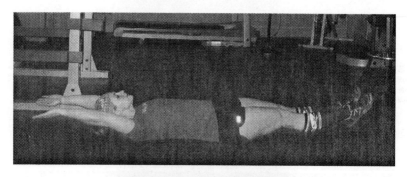

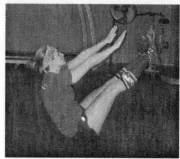

V-ups

Home-made equipment

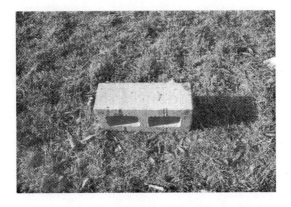

Stone used for landscaping from a home improvement store

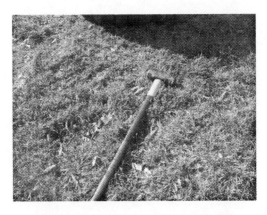

Sledgehammer purchased from a home improvement store. They vary in weight and size.

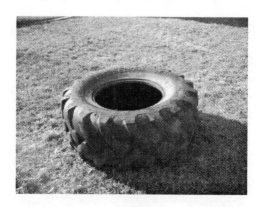

Used Tire from my dad's garage, Anytime Truck and Tire in Altoona, PA

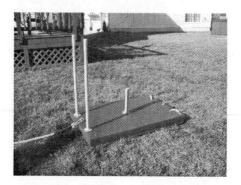

Home-made Sled

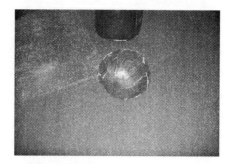

Home-made Medicine Ball (dodge ball, sand and duct tape)

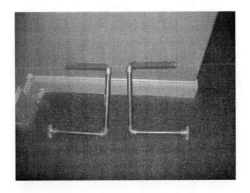

Farmer's Walk, plumbers piping screwed together

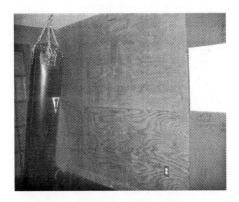

Plywood hung on a wall

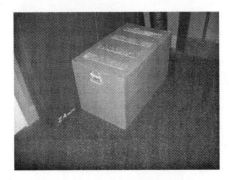

Home-made box used for box jumps or as a bench

Workouts sans equipment or with home-made equipment

Any of these exercises can be substituted for a different exercise depending on your fitness level, or if you are injured. If you cannot do push-ups then do knee push-ups or wall push-ups. If you cannot sprint then jog or walk. I have had super-obese clients complete the work-outs below. They are for **EVERYBODY**.

If you are just starting out you can start scaling the workout by timing yourself. Set a timer for 12 minutes and complete as much of the work out as you can in those 12 minutes. Do not be afraid to take breaks and/or drink water, but keep them as brief as possible.

If you cannot do an exercise in the full range of motion, for instance you cannot get your hips down low for a squat; you go as low as you can. If you cannot drop your shoulders down for a dip; then you go as low as you can. The only person you are competing against is you! Just don't quit!

Day One, Week One

5x5 (5 rounds of 5 repetitions)

Squat

Burpee

Walking lunge (5 steps each leg)

Burpee

After this circuit do 100 sit-ups (just one set!)

Day Two, Week One

Shuttle Run. Pick about 50 yards distance. Race back and forth (25 yards) and touch your hand to the ground and then race back to the start line three times.

After the Shuttle Runs are complete do 50 hand release push-ups.

112

Day Three, Week One

A rep scheme of 20, 15, 10 (three rounds total; you will do 20 repetitions the first round, 15 repetitions the second round and 10 repetitions the last round)

Dips

Plank Get-outs

Box Jumps (step up and down if you can't make the jump yet....eventually you will)

Day Four, Week One

Set a timer for 12 minutes and do as many rounds as you possibly can in those 12 minutes of the following exercises:

10 squats, 10 push-ups, 10 dips and 10 jumping jacks

10 repetitions of each of the four exercises counts as one round, then you start over until the 12 minute buzzer goes off; try to take as few breaks as possible.

Day Five, Week One

HIIT Jumping Jacks!

Using a timer do jumping jacks for 30 seconds; rest for 20 seconds and then right back into the jumping jacks. Do this for eight rounds.

Day Six, Week One

30 minute walk – active recovery

Day Seven, Week One

Complete each stretch in the Stretching Section holding each stretch for at least 30 seconds.

**Add in rest days as you need – if you need more rest days than annotated....take them!!

Day One, Week Two

A 300!

100 sit-ups

100 push-ups

100 squats

Day Two, Week Two

6 rounds of

20 repetitions of mountain climbers

Run in place (knees hip high) for 20 seconds

6 repetitions of Parkour push-ups

Day Three, Week Two

Waiter Lunge x 100 steps

Day Four, Week Two

10, 50 yard Sprints

10, 50 yard Skipping (yep, just like you did when you are a kid! HIGH KNEES!)

Day Five, Week Two

6 rounds of 6 repetitions each

Burpees

Pike Push-ups

Jumps

Spider Kicks (6 each side)

Day Six, Week Two

30 minute walk active recovery

Day Seven, Week Two

Stretching, active recovery

Day One, Week Three

2 minutes of each exercise with a 1 minute rest in between for 2 rounds.

Bunny Hops

Bear Crawl

Sit ups

Day Two, Week Three

3 rounds of 2 minutes with 1 minute rest in between each round.

Farmer's Walk 50 yards

Yoke Walk 50 yards

Sprint back to Farmer's Walk's equipment

Stage gear for Yoke Walk 50 yards from start. Begin with Farmer's Walk down to Yoke Walk's staged gear. Drop Farmer's Walk's gear and pick up Yoke Walk's gear and walk back to start line. Drop Yoke Walk's gear and sprint back to Farmer's Walk's gear. Repeat for 2 minutes. Do this for 3 rounds.

Day Three, Week Three

A 500! For time

100 mountain climbers

25 plank get outs

25 sit-ups

25 spider kicks

25 v-ups

100 dips

100 squats

Day Four, Week Three

6 rounds of 6 repetitions

Hip thrusts

Kneeling Get-ups

Un-weighted overhead squats

Bridges

Scoot

Shrimp

Day Five, Week Three

100 Burpees for time

Day Five, Week Three

30 minute walk active recovery

Day Five, Week Three

Stretching, active recovery

Equipment based workouts

Day One, Week One

2 repetitions to failure of Dead Lift

5x5 @ 75% of Dead Lift

Then….

2 repetitions of each exercise for 12 rounds

Pull-ups, Barbell Curls (100% max weight), Dumbbell Row (100% max weight) chin-ups

Day Two, Week One

21, 18, 15, 12, 9, 6, 3 (for time)

Dumb Bell Bench Press (start light in weight and go heavier as repetitions decrease)

Box Jumps

Hand Release Push-ups

Sit-ups

Day Three, Week One

30 minute walk active recovery

Day Four, Week One

5x10 @ 55-65 % max weight

Shoulder Barbell Press

Front Squat

Front and Side Lateral Raises

Stiff Leg Dead Lift

Abs Roll Out

Day Five, Week One

75 Dips

.25 mile sprint

50 Kickbacks (50 each arm)

.25 mile sprint

25 Pull-ups

Day Six, Week One

30 minute walk active recovery

Day Seven

Stretch active recovery

Day One, Week Two

2 to fail and 5x5 @ 75% Back Squat

Then....

One round of 25 repetitions of each exercise; no resting between exercise and sprint.

Hip Thrusts

Sprint .25mile

Hand Release Push-ups

Sprint .25 mile

Hyperextensions

Sprint .25 mile

Plank get-outs

Sprint .25 mile

Day Two, Week Two

One round of 25 repetitions of each exercise

Skull Crushers @ 55-65% of max

.25 mile sprint

Rocky Presses (50% max of shoulder press)

.25 mile sprint

Chin ups

.25 mile sprint

Pull ups

.25 mile sprint

Day Three, Week Two

30 minute walk active recovery

Day Four, Week Two

20, 15, 10, 5 repetitions of

Bench Press @ 55-65% of max

Burpees

Sit-ups

Day Five, Week Two

7 rounds of 7 repetitions of each exercise at 60% of max for weights

Barbell Row with Drop Dead Stop

Rear Deltoid Fly

Shrimp

Wall Ball or an Explosive Push-ups if no equipment for wall ball

Day Six, Week Two

30 minute walk for active recovery

Day Seven, Week Two

Stretching for active recovery

Day One, Week Three

2 to fail and 5x5 @ 75% Push Press

Then.....

3 rounds

10 Front/Side Lateral Raises

10 Dumbbell Rows

100 Jump Rope revolutions

Day Two, Week Three

3 rounds

5 Dead Lift, 5 Bench Press, and 6 Burpees

Do these 3 exercises back to back with little to no rest in between each exercise. Then rest for 2 minutes. Repeat for 3 rounds.

Complete these exercises with 50% your max weight going slow into it and exploding out. For example on the Deadlift go slow into the down position and explode up! PROPER FORM!!!! It's not about the weight it's about the explosion and the form.

Day Three, Week Three

30 minute active recovery walks

Day Four, Week Three

3 rounds

5 Barbell Row w/ dead stop, 5 Back Squat, 6 Burpees

Circuit fashion same as Day Two of this week; same 50% max weight and same slow into the movement with an explosive out.

Day Five, Week Three

A 500! For time

100 mountain climbers

25 plank get outs

25 sit-ups

25 spider kicks

25 v-ups

100 dips

100 squats

Day Six, Week Three

30 minute active recovery walk

Day Seven, Week Three

Stretching for active recover

Day One, Week Four

Complete the following exercises for each of the following repetition and weight schematics.

	55% x 5	65% x 5	75% x 1	85% x 1	95% x 1	85% x 3
Back Squat						
Dead Lift						
Push Press						

Day Two, Week Four

Walk and stretch for active recovery

Day Three, Week Four

A 300!

100 sit-ups

100 push-ups

100 squats

Day Four, Week Four

2 repetitions to failure of Bench Press

5x5 @ 75% of max Bench Press

100 sit-ups

Day Five, Week Four

6 rounds of 6 repetitions

Bridges

Front and Side Lateral Raises

Hip Thrusts

Kneeling Get-up

100 jump rope at the end of each round

Day Six, Week Four

Walk for 30 minutes active recovery

Day Seven, Week Four

Stretch for active recovery

STRETCHES

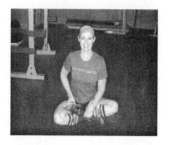

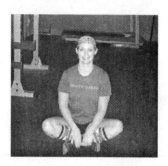

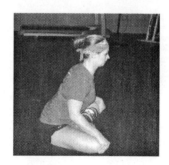

Hip Flexors

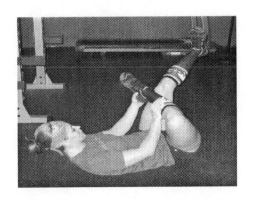

Illotibial Band

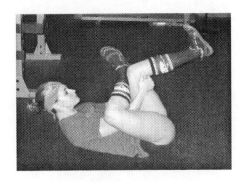

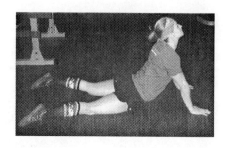

Lower Back

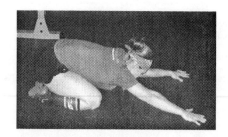

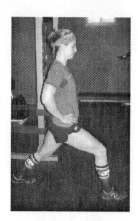

Achilles tendon

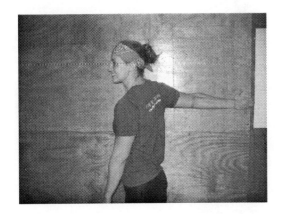
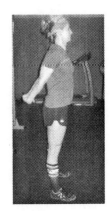

Shoulder

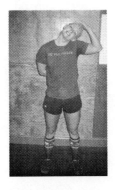

Neck

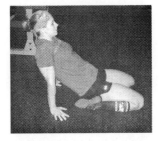

Quadriceps

Chapter Seven:

Recipes

Please note that I am a lazy chef and use the "eyeball technique" as my measuring. I always use coconut oil to grease to cook with. All the beef I use is grass-fed beef and the only sweetener I use is honey (and extremely sparingly). Get creative and have fun!

Breakfast

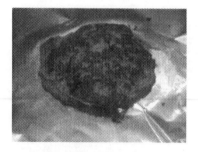

Pancakes

1/2 c unsweetened applesauce or unsweetened pumpkin

4 Tbsp Cashew Butter or Almond Butter

2 eggs

Cinnamon to taste

1 Tbsp Vanilla

Mix all ingredients. Grill on low to medium heat. Coconut oil to grease pan. You can also take this same mix and put into mini cupcake liners and bake until set for mini muffins. Be creative and add berries to the mix or slivers of dark chocolate.

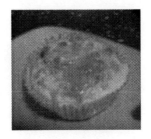

Egg Quiche

8 oz cream cheese

8 eggs

Chopped meat if you desire (ham, sausage, bacon)

Veggies of your choice (green pepper, onion)

Garlic, pepper, salt

Whip. Pour into greased pie pan or divide in cupcake pan. Bake at 325 degrees until center is slightly wiggly. Pull out of oven and let sit. The eggs will continue to cook once out of the oven. If you cook until it is solid it will be dry and rubbery.

Apple Scrambler

5 eggs

2 apples cubed

Cinnamon

Walnut oil for skillet

Walnuts

Brown apples in skillet with walnut, cinnamon and walnut oil. Add in eggs. Scramble. (Can substitute apples and walnuts with peaches and pecans)

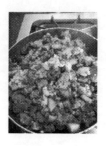

Kitchen Sink!

Nitrate Free Sausage

Red Potatoes

Eggs

Green Pepper and Onion (if you want)

Garlic, Pepper, Salt

Cut red potatoes into cubes (how many depends on how many people you are trying to feed and if you want leftovers). Cook potatoes on the stove in a skillet with coconut oill or butter, garlic, pepper and salt. Add in green peppers and onions when potatoes are almost complete. Potatoes are done when tender to a fork. Brown sausage (again how much depends on how much you are trying to make) in a separate skillet and add to cooked potatoes. Cook eggs and scramble (how many eggs depends on you!) in separate skillet and when done add to potatoes and sausage.

Dinner

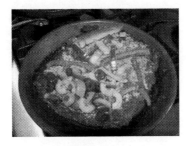

Meatsa Pizza

Package of nitrate-free sausage or beef

Veggies of your choice

Tomato sauce

Press sausage into a pie pan and bake until brown. Sautee veggies on the stove. Be creative. Add garlic, onion, Italian seasonings, peppers, olives – make it flavorful! Spread sauce over meat and top with veggies.

Steak Chili:

12 oz thinly sliced round steak
1 large green, red, yellow pepper diced
1/2 cup diced onion

½ c cranberries
1 can diced green chilies (4.5 oz)
9 Jalapeno pepper slices (diced)
14 oz can diced tomatoes (slightly drained)
1 tsp. cumin

Spray nonstick pan with cooking spray. Cook beef fully. Add remaining ingredients. Simmer covered 20 minutes. Simmer uncovered 20-30 minutes (until desired consistency).

Meat Loaf

Beef
1 egg
3/4 cup coconut milk
1/2 small onion, minced

1 tbsp Dijon mustard

¼ tomato paste
1/2 teaspoon hot pepper sauce (or 1 tsp rooster sauce)
1.5 tablespoons Worcestershire sauce
1/4 teaspoon ground black pepper

Spices of your choice

Heat oven to 350. Mix ingredients. Place in a baking dish. Bake 35 minutes or until center is set.

Spicy Thai Chicken
1 1/2 pound boneless, skinless chicken breasts, cut in chunks
1 medium red and green bell pepper, cut into strips
3 tbsp almond butter

1/4 c. honey

2 TBSP Lime or Lemon Juice

Coconut Oil
1 tsp (I put 1 tbsp) Thai-style red curry paste
1 tbsp chopped green onion

Directions
Coat wok or nonstick frying pan with coconut oil. Sauté the chicken add ingredients – heat and serve.

Turkey sausage and eggplant lasagna

1 lb eggplant
1.25 lbs ground turkey
1 tbsp. red pepper flake
.5 cup onion, chopped
.5 cup bell pepper, chopped
4 cloves garlic, chopped
1 cup canned chopped tomatoes

1 tbsp. chopped fresh oregano
1 tbsp. chopped fresh basil
2 eggs
1 tbsp. chopped parsley
salt and pepper to taste

Preheat oven to 350 degrees. Peel and thinly slice eggplant. Arrange in one layer on baking sheet and bake until tender. Meanwhile, sauté garlic, onion, bell pepper, red pepper flake in nonstick skillet coated with cooking spray until soft. Season with salt and pepper. Put in a bowl and mix eggs into veggies. Add turkey and brown until cooked through. Season with salt and pepper. Add chopped tomato and a bit of water and simmer for ~20 minutes. Add basil and oregano stir through and season with salt and pepper to taste.

Assemble by spreading .25 cup sauce in bottom of baking pan. Add a single layer of eggplant, followed by a layer of sauce mixture. Layer casserole until all ingredients are used or baking dish is full. Cover and bake on 350 for ~20 minutes.

Stuffed Peppers

You can use red or yellow peppers but they need to stand up on their own.
6 large bell peppers
1 lb. lean ground beef
1/2 cup chopped onion
2 cups broccoli
1 can (15oz) tomato sauce (I like to buy the tomato, garlic, basil flavored)
1/4 tsp garlic powder or more for taste
1 tsp salt more or less for taste
You can chop up any other veggies too if you like and throw them in.

Heat oven to 350 degrees. Cut thin holes out of top of pepper and remove stems, and seeds. Cook and stir ground beef with onion or any other veggies you are throwing in. Drain beef mixture. Stir in salt, garlic, rice, and only 1 cup of the tomato sauce; heat through.
Lightly stuff each pepper to the top with the meat mixture. Stand peppers upright in an ungreased baking dish (8x8x2). Pour remaining tomato sauce

over tops of peppers. Cover with foil and bake for 20 minutes. Uncover and bake for 15 more minutes. You can sprinkle some low fat cheddar cheese on them and bake for the last 5 minutes if you like.

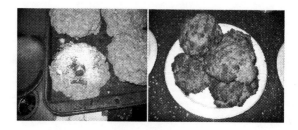

Wolf Burgers

Ground meat your choice

Veggies and cheese

Seasonings

Mold meat into patties. Add veggies and cheese to center of patties and top with another patties. Pinch edges. Grill.

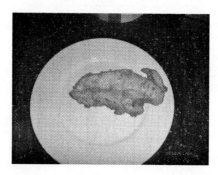

Fried Chicken or Tilapia

Chicken Breasts or Tilapia

Coconut Flour

Garlic Salt

Eggs

Coconut Oil

Beat eggs. Combine coconut flour and garlic salt. Dip chicken breasts in egg and then in coconut flour mixture. On low to medium heat coconut oil and drop coated chicken breast into oil. Fry for about eight minutes.

Lime and Mustard Chicken

1 lb skinless, boneless chicken breasts
½ cup fresh lime juice
½ cup fresh cilantro, chopped
¼ cup Dijon mustard
1 tablespoon olive oil
1 tablespoon chili powder
½ tsp salt
½ tsp pepper

Combine lime juice, cilantro, mustard, olive oil, chili, salt and pepper in a food processor. Pulse until ingredients are well combined. Rinse chicken breasts, pat dry and place in a 7x11 inch Pyrex baking dish. Pour marinade over chicken, cover and refrigerate for at least 15 minutes or up to 6 hours. Heat grill and cook chicken for 5-7 minutes per side until browned and cooked in the center. Serves two.

Mexican Chicken and "Rice"
Coconut oil
1 medium onion, diced
1 cup celery, finely diced
1 head cauliflower, trimmed
1 (4 ounce) can green chilies, diced
1 pound boneless, skinless chicken breast, grilled and diced into 1-inch pieces
1 tsp salt
ground cumin, oregano and chili powder to taste
1 avocado
grated cheese, if desired
salsa, if desired

In a large skillet, heat coconut oil over medium heat. Sauté onion over medium heat for 10 minutes, until soft. Add celery to skillet and sauté for 5 minutes. Place cauliflower in a food processor with the "S" blade and process until the texture of rice. Add cauliflower to skillet, cover and cook 5-10 minutes, until soft. Mix chilies and chicken into skillet. Stir in salt, cumin, oregano and chili powder. Serve, topping with avocado, cheese and salsa if desired.

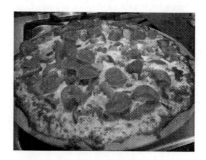

Cauliflower Crust Pizza

4 cups cauliflower ground like rice in food processor

3 eggs

2.5 c shredded cheese

Italian seasonings

Mix and arrange on a cooking stone or cookie sheet in pizza shape. Cook at 450 degrees for 25 minutes.

Add toppings as desired and put back in oven on broil for 3-4 minutes.

Shrimp Cakes

1 pound (raw) shrimp, peeled and deveined

1 red or yellow bell pepper, finely chopped

1 clove garlic, minced

2 tablespoons scallions, thinly sliced

1 tablespoon lime juice

1 tablespoon honey

½ teaspoon salt

¼ teaspoon chipotle seasoning

1 egg

½ cup cilantro, finely chopped

½ cup blanched almond flour

3 tablespoons coconut oil, for sautéing

Place shrimp in food processor, pulse until finely chopped. In a large bowl, combine chopped shrimp, bell pepper, garlic, scallions, lime juice, honey, salt, chipotle, egg and cilantro. Form mixture into patties, dip each in almond flour, coating thoroughly. In a large skillet, over medium heat, warm 1 tablespoon oil. Add to the skillet and cook about 5 minutes per side, until browned; remove and place on paper towel lined plate. Makes 12.

Side Dishes

<u>Mashed Cauliflower (like mashed potatoes)</u>

Boil whole cauliflower in water for 30 minutes or until tender. In a casserole dish mash with fork. Add 2 TBSP Butter. Lemon pepper to taste.

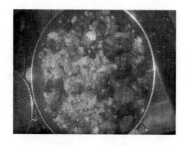

<u>Fried "Rice" Cauliflower(shown w/ grass-fed beef kilbasa)</u>

Coconut Oil

Garlic

Salt

Cauliflower

With a serrated knife cut cauliflower in a sawing motion. The cauliflower will cut off like rice. In a skillet with the rest of the ingredients cook until brown.

<u>Potato Salad</u>

Red potatoes

Mayo

Celery

Onions

Hard Boiled Eggs

Boil potatoes in skin until skin peels off. You can live skin on or peel off. Cut potatoes and eggs into cubes. Cut celery and onions into slivers. Mix potatoes, celery and onion with mayo.

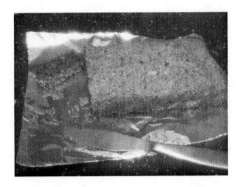

Simple Bread

2 ½ cups blanched almond flour (or grind your own nuts in a food processor! This loaf pictured was made with walnuts. It comes out darker than when made with almonds)

½ teaspoon salt

½ teaspoon baking soda

3 eggs

1 tablespoon honey

½ teaspoon apple cider vinegar

In a large bowl, combine almond flour, salt and baking soda. In a medium bowl, whisk the eggs, add honey and vinegar. Stir wet ingredients into dry. Scoop batter into a well greased 6.5 x 4 inch baby loaf pan. (Double recipe for regular loaf pan). Bake at 300° for 45-55 minutes on bottom rack of oven; until a knife comes out clean. Cool and serve

Onion Rings

Coconut Oil

Almond Flour

Egg

Big yellow onions

In a deep pot heat coconut oil (not a running boil). Slice onion into rings. Dip in beat egg. Dip in almond flour. Re-dip in egg and almond flour. Drop into pot and brown.

Sweet Potato Chips

Sweet Potatoes

Cinnamon

Salt

Grease a cookie sheet. Heat oven to 375 degrees. Slice sweet potato into ¼ inch slices. Sprinkle with salt and cinnamon and bake for 40 minutes or until desired crispness.

Potato Chips

Red Potatoes

Salt

Grease cookie sheet. Heat oven to 375 degrees. Slice red potatoes into ¼ inch or thinner slices and sprinkle with salt. Bake for 40 minutes or until desired crispness.

Stuffing (Same as Kitchen Sink breakfast without eggs!)

4 red skinned potatoes

1 package of sausage

Celery, onion

Italian seasoning

Cut potatoes into small cubes. Brown in a skillet with butter. Add in sausage and continue to break sausage into small bits as it cooks. Chop celery and onion to slivers and mix in.

Treats

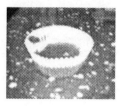

Cashew butter melts

1 box unsweetened cacao squares

12 Mini muffin liners

12 tsp. Cashew butter or Almond butter

Honey

Heat chocolate in a microwave safe container or double-boiler on the stove until melted (do not boil chocolate) add in honey – the amount of honey is determined by how sweet YOU want it. I only use about ¼ c. but I like my chocolate bitter.

Fill mini muffin liner half full. Add a tsp. of cashew or almond butter and cover with chocolate and refrigerate.

Paleo Ice Cream

3 c Unsweetened Almond or Coconut Milk

1/3 c honey

1/3 c cocoa powder

2 tbsp vanilla

1 tsp. xanthium gum

Mix ingredients in blender on whip. Pour into ice cream maker. You can also make plain vanilla by leaving out the cocoa powder. Or add in fruit or different extracts (like mint with chunks of chocolate for mint chocolate chip). Be creative!

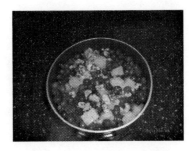

Cranberry and pineapple sauce

3 c. Fresh cranberries

1 pineapple cut into chunks (or 2 seedless oranges)

3 c water

Walnuts (optional)

½ c honey

Boil cranberries and oranges in 3 c water. Cook until cranberries pop. Take off heat. Add walnuts and honey and let cool and thicken.

Fudge

1 package Baker's square cacao

2 c heavy whipping cream

½ c honey

1 tsp salt

Walnuts

Boil ingredients on stove or in a microwave. Place in greased dish and refrigerate.

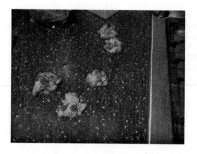

Chocolate Chip Cookies

4c. Almond Flour

1 c. honey

1 tsp each salt, baking soda, baking powder

½ c each 53% or higher dark chocolate chips and 100% chocolate in small pieces

4 eggs

2 tsp Vanilla extract

Pre-heat oven to 375 degrees. Mix ingredients, drop batter in spoonful on to greased cookie sheet. Bake for 12 minutes.

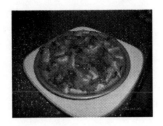

Cheesecake

Crust:

2 c. walnuts or almonds crushed

1 egg

¼ c butter

Mix and press into pie pan. Bake for 10 minutes at 325 degrees.

Cake:

8 oz cream cheese

2 tsp vanilla extract

3 eggs

¼ c honey

Mix together and pour in pie shell and bake at 325 degrees for 40 minutes. Put in fridge.

Apple Crisp

In greased pie pan cut in slices 5 Apples of your choice add cinnamon.

Crisp:

1 c unsweetened coconut flakes

¼ c butter

Chopped walnuts

145

½ c almond flour

Cinnamon

Melt butter, mix ingredients and crumble over apples. Bake at 350 degrees covered with foil for 20 minutes. Bake another 10 minutes without foil to brown crumble.

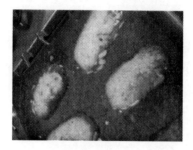

__Almond Biscotti__

3 c. Almond Flour

2 TBSP Almond Extract

½ c. Almond Oil

4 Eggs

1 TBSP Baking Powder

1 TSP Salt

½ c. Honey

100% Chocolate Squares

Mix all ingredients except chocolate. Line a bread pan with parchment paper. Bake at 375 degrees for 25 minutes. Pull out. Cool. Cut and put back into oven for 10 minutes (or until crunchy). Cool. Heat chocolate squares in microwavable bowl and "paint" a thin coat of chocolate on the edge.